MAKING THE CASE FOR YOURSELF

Making the Case for Yourself

A Diet Book for Smart Women

SUSAN ESTRICH

RIVERHEAD BOOKS

a member of

Penguin Putnam Inc.

New York

1998

RIVERHEAD BOOKS
a member of
Penguin Putnam Inc.
200 Madison Avenue
New York, NY 10016

Library of Congress Cataloging-in-Publication Data

Estrich, Susan.
Making the case for yourself : a diet book for smart women / by Susan Estrich.
p.   cm.
ISBN 1-57322-083-3
1. Weight loss.   I. Title.
RM222.2.E88   1998   97-35494 CIP
613.2'5—dc21

Printed in the United States of America
1   3   5   7   9   10   8   6   4   2
This book is printed on acid-free paper. ∞

Book design by Ralph Fowler

ACKNOWLEDGMENTS

Amanda Urban thought it was a good idea,
but the best idea was Julie Grau.

*To Marty, Isabel, James,
and Mr. Hershey Kaplan*

CONTENTS

MAKING THE CASE FOR YOURSELF

You're Writing a What?

For at least the last twenty years, I've been struck by a very central contradiction in my life. I could do almost any task I set for myself. Except one.

Lose weight.

I have worked when I was exhausted, dealt with people who are impossible, situations which were intractable, I've dragged myself out of bed when I could barely see straight to take responsibility for things I hadn't even done.

I can do all that, and then I can't resist a poor old dried-up danish?

I can't. Or at least I couldn't.

I spent twenty-five years smashing my head against glass ceilings and breaking through more than once. But I always stopped for the danish. And I hated myself for it.

I was the first woman president of the Harvard Law Review, the first woman to run a presidential campaign, and a tenured professor at Harvard Law School at thirty-three. I clerked on the United States Supreme Court and worked for the chief counsel of the Senate Judiciary Committee. I've written three books about the criminal justice system, including one in which I used my own experience as a rape victim as a basis to argue for reform. I go on national television all the time, taking on defense lawyers and conservatives and even the Speaker of the House; I write a syndicated column twice a week, and teach law and political science at USC, and serve on the board of my kids' school. But nothing I do now or have done in the past (other than falling in love with the right guy, and having our children, which I consider blessings, not accomplishments) has made me prouder, happier, or more fulfilled than losing weight and getting in shape.

I have been a size 6 (sometimes a 4) for three years now, and I spent all the ones before that between 10 and 14, mostly closer to 14. I lift weights, do push-ups, wear sleeveless dresses, and wave at the beach. I was in a dressing room not long ago, trying on jean shorts just for the fun of it (imagine that), when a young saleswoman walked by, saw me looking in the mirror and said, "What a cute figure you have." I looked around to make sure it was me she was talking to; no one had said that to me since I went away to college. I feel as if I've finally checked this piece of excess baggage that I've been dragging around for decades. My only regret is that I didn't do it sooner.

For twenty-three years—but who's counting—I was on a diet, about to start a diet, or breaking a diet. For twenty-three years, I went up and down and up and down, lying to myself, putting myself down, demanding the impossible and failing even to get close. For twenty-three years, I dreaded shopping, three-way mirrors, the weight question on my license, and seeing pictures of myself.

Over those years, I've bought almost every diet book written, searching far and wide for that holy grail—the diet that would make me thin. I have been on smart diets, stupid diets, healthy diets, and downright dangerous ones. I have eaten only protein, and no protein; only carbohydrates, and no carbohydrates; carbohydrates and protein together, and carbohydrates and protein separately. I have tried food combinations, liquid brews, frozen food, dehydrated food, group diets, and one-on-one diets. I have joined the weekly clubs and signed up for daily check-ins. I have spent money I didn't have joining programs I couldn't afford, buying exercise equipment I didn't use, and ordering videos I rarely played.

No matter what I was doing or how much pressure I was under, I've gotten up every morning and stepped on the scale. Before the days of digital scales, I'd lean to one side and look from the other. When the reading was "bad," my reaction would be simple. I'd hate myself. I allowed my weight to determine my attitude for the day; I have let it turn good days into bad ones.

Of course I knew this was stupid. Being a size 14 American woman is not like being a refugee in a war-torn land. But being told, even by yourself, that you should not feel as bad as you do does not make you feel better; it only makes you eat. A "bad" day on the morning scale for me would usually turn into one in which I ate too much, not too little.

Stuck in the vicious cycle, I tried to convince myself that the problem wasn't my body but my attitude, and that if only I could rid myself of these harmful and sexist attitudes that celebrate slim women with strong bodies, then I'd be fine. I read all the popular books by beautiful feminists that were supposed to convince you that being slim and beautiful is just some sexist man's fantasy, but frankly, on me the books failed. They don't liberate me. I don't look in the mirror and smile at my stomach. I don't feel better about my body. I just feel vain, foolish, and stupid in addition to fat.

I don't want to convince you that looking good is a slightly foolish obsession that properly centered, successful women can ill afford. I want to convince you of just the opposite.

Of course the quest for slimness can be taken to an extreme, particularly when looking good is divorced from feeling good and being healthy. But so can any quest. Most of us who are chronic diet failures are in no danger of being too thin. The challenge is to be our best, and that includes looking our best, in the eyes of others and ourselves.

I think being slim and healthy and sexy and feeling great about yourself are actually positive attitudes, and a tremendous source of potential power for women. I don't aspire to look like Kate Moss; I don't aspire to being as smart as Einstein either, but that's no excuse for not being my best.

Why, asked one of my friends, when she heard I was writing a diet book, aren't you writing a book about something serious, something important, something worthy? She thinks people should use their brains to their best ability, and focus on what's important. So do I.

So I told her. I am doing something important. I'm writing a diet book.

My reasons for writing this book were partly selfish. I don't mean that I was looking for money, which I'm certainly happy to find. I mean that I was worried about myself.

I worked for one of the networks as an "expert" during the first O. J. Simpson trial, which meant I was on television during endless sidebars, and as a result, was often recognized in the street, at the market, in dressing rooms. Wherever I went in Los Angeles, before anyone would bring up the Simpson case, they'd ask me an even more pressing question. How did you do it? How did you lose all that weight?

Here I was, thin for the first time in my life, on television all the time, feeling better about myself than I ever had before. But sometimes at night, I'd have dreams in which I was fat again, and wake up to reassure myself that my spare tire was still gone.

I knew what I had done to lose weight; I'd done it, after all, on my own this time. But it wasn't just the women who sidled up to me in dressing rooms who needed answers. I needed them, too. Had I really changed? How? Could I pull this business of dieting together the way I would master, say, a new area of law, and make it mine?

My second year of teaching, I was asked to teach labor law. It was a perfectly reasonable request, except for the fact that I knew no labor law; I'd never taken a course in it, never practiced in the field, and while I'd spent a fair amount of my time in union halls doing politics, I had never actually sat down and read the National Labor Relations Act. "No better way to learn a course than to teach it," one of my senior colleagues told me. I taught labor law, and in the process, taught it to myself.

That's what I decided to do with dieting, with the advantage that here I started with a track record of twenty-something years, amazingly enough capped by success. I had done "it." Now all I had to do was figure out what "it" was with enough clarity that I could write a book that would help others do "it" too. And help me never gain it back.

How long does it take before you really know you're thin, I asked one friend, who's been a size 6 since I knew her, but was a size 14 for a couple of decades before that. Five years, she told me. In my case, it took a book.

"How did you do it?" I was asked time and again, across lines of age and race and ethnic origin, from good friends to casual acquaintances, from Hillary Clinton to the ladies in the Loehmann's dressing room.

Translate: How did you go from being a 140-pound blob—well, maybe 152 on a bad day, but who's counting—to having this great body now attached to a familiar head?

And, unstated but overarching, "Can I do it too?"

You can.

The women who would approach me in restaurants, at dinner parties, at the grocery store were all smart, competent women, who could tell you how to run a school or a business, manage money, sell a house, organize a fundraiser. But when it comes to dieting we throw common sense to the wind, taking pills we wouldn't feed to our puppies, going on diets so ridiculous we often don't want to admit it to our own friends. We are desperate for someone to tell us a secret, willing to try anything that we haven't already failed at, willing to listen to anyone who tells us they can make us thin. And we fail, over and over again.

I used to think of dieting as an act of willpower, exercising a muscle, almost like lifting a weight. You grunt your way to the full contraction, breathing through the pain, Lamaze as life. Going on a diet was an act of planned deprivation, intentional pain; sticking to it involved forcing myself, almost physically, not to reach for the brownie, stop for the ice cream, head for the cookies in frustration. It was all about forcing myself not to do what I desperately wanted to do. I could pull it off for a while, a day, a week, the two months before my wedding. But who could do it forever? Not me.

Here's the truth: The key to the success of my last diet was that I stuck to it. What changed most profoundly was my attitude. I trained myself to think differently. I cheated less. I constantly reminded myself of what I was doing and why I was doing it. I fulfilled my intentions, stood up to temptation, separated eating from all the other functions it served, and ate less. I tapped into my skills as a lawyer and a teacher and turned them on myself. I developed an arsenal of arguments capable of being deployed on a moment's notice to remind my grabbing hands of just why I was on a diet, and what I hoped to accomplish, and how the muffin was probably stale anyway. I made the case for my diet. And it worked.

But that is not what the women at the grocery store want to hear, even if they know it's the truth, and it's probably not what you're looking for right now. You want a diet. You want a secret. You want something that will work magic in three days, let you feast for a week, let you eat everything in sight for as long as you want, and still lose weight. You want a miracle.

Why is that? Why do we search for miracle cures when Western medicine can tell you how to lose weight? Why are we willing to suspend better judgment, something we're unwilling to do in every other aspect of life, when it comes to our very well-being? Why is it that professional women can be so totally competent when it comes to taking care of business, and can't even see what terrible care we're taking of ourselves? Why do intelligent women get stupid when it comes to their own bodies?

We run our lives like adults, and diet like teenagers. The excuses we come up with make my friends in the criminal defense bar look like advocates of strict liability. *I work so hard, I'm so tired, it's my only pleasure, it doesn't really count, because I deserve it so, and besides, I'm going on a diet tomorrow.* A miracle diet.

I'll never stop you from being stupid about diets just by telling you you're being stupid. Who wants another sensible book that tells you to eat fruit and vegetables? You know the food groups. You want a miracle. I know that. I was you for most of my life.

I have good news. You've come to the right place. I sat down and approached diets like the A student I am and decided to break the code. Surely I could impose order on the hundreds of diet books on my desk, and the dozens of diets I'd gone on and made up myself in the process of losing my weight. We all know that in the end we have to take responsibility for the way we eat, but in the beginning we're desperate for someone else to assume it. How do you get from the beginning to the end in real terms, not just with words? Is there anything connecting the different piles of books, any logic to this topsy-turvy world that has run my life as much as the federal code of law?

I think I cracked it. I devised four diets. You go on them in order. It's a sequence that takes you from listening to me to listening to yourself. You will lose weight fast. It will almost be easy. You will never be hungry. You will never be bored. I have a Three-Day Wonder Diet, a Five-Day Feast, and an All-You-Can-Eat Diet. I have devoted thirty years of my life and whatever intellectual gifts God gave me to the pursuit of the perfect diet, and I think I finally figured it out. Your internist might smirk as if he knows better, and then ask you for my recipe for cabbage soup.

Yes, Virginia, there *is* a diet.

Do you feel better now?

Good. I thought you would.

I decided to call it "Susan's Miracle Diet," because I wouldn't want it to feel out of place at the bookstore or in the library.

I'll tell you all its secrets just as soon as we negotiate the terms of your commitment and I get your signature on the bottom line of the contract. Remember, I'm a lawyer. I have a diet. But we need to strike a deal, you and me. Because you have the power to make it work or break the deal.

You know the mindset you use to succeed—the smart, competent woman who pulls off the near-impossible every day. The one who gets up in the night, finds the Motrin, takes care of the kid with the fever, gets out of bed again three hours later to get the other one ready for school and to get to work yourself, where you keep six balls in the air, while you have the drugstore on hold trying to find the prescription the pediatrician called in. You know this woman.

What if she went on a diet?

If you can do three things at the same time, while juggling a life and a job and your own family and your civic group and the needs of everyone and everything else in the world, I'm here to tell you, you *can* resist a dried-up danish.

Don't kid yourself. You won't be able to do any of those other things if you don't take better care of yourself. You come in with your body and you go out with it. When it stops working, so do you. If you don't take care of it, it's liable to wear out before you do. I know many people who take better care of their cars than they do of themselves, who worry about flying on planes when they ought to be worrying about sitting down at the dinner table with their kids. We think of ourselves as smart women, and yet we treat our bodies as our enemies instead of our single greatest assets, a living miracle that we trash.

There is nothing you can do that would be a bigger gift for yourself and your family than to lose weight and get in shape. It can save your life, your marriage, your sense of self-esteem. You won't lose weight unless you believe that. Fortunately, it's true.

I'm a teacher. I teach law, which is to say I teach people a certain way to think. People who aren't lawyers assume that there is this mass of rules—the law—which you learn when you go to law school. It should be so easy. Oh, there are statutes and past decisions, which are supposed to guide your decision, but in the hard cases we teach, there are always two sides. What you really learn to do is make a case, structure an argument, anticipate objections, and lay them to rest in advance.

The method is tried and tested. The professor, à la the famed

Kingsfield in *The Paper Chase,* asks question after question, following one side's argument and then the other's, demanding that you answer points you can barely believe you were lucky enough to see, and explain decisions you took for granted. You remain on the hook until all the brain muscle you have has been expended in taking apart and analyzing whatever tiny nugget that's being used to make the point. It's a process that, when it works, changes the way you think, and that change is the most lasting part of your legal education. There's that voice in your head pushing you on to make the argument stronger, pointing out every logical inconsistency you were trying to slip by, pulling you back from the conclusion to show you what you've taken for granted, the piece of the argument you have not answered. It's what people mean when they say that you "think like a lawyer": you know how to frame a case, how to put together an argument, how to find the jugular and win. It is a skill that is probably more highly regarded than the profession it is attached to.

I met the man who became my husband when I was working for Geraldine Ferraro and he was working for former Vice-President Walter Mondale. After the Democratic Convention, when my boss was selected as the vice-presidential nominee, I turned down a chance at a very senior job in her operation with all my friends from Massachusetts so that I could take a drudge job on the Mondale plane, and sit next to my new boyfriend for four months instead of never seeing him. It was the year my older sister, then thirty-three, was diagnosed with cancer, which certainly figured in my decision. Gerry understood, in a way most male bosses probably would not have; putting personal life first isn't something most men do, which is their loss.

I sat behind the candidate, in the window seat, where it's hard to get out, so you just eat all the time. And listen. Whenever there was a difficult issue to be resolved, Mondale would say,

"We need Arthur Liman to make the case . . ." The late Arthur Liman was one of America's most distinguished lawyers, then practicing in New York, and rarely available in mid-flight to structure the argument. What Mr. Mondale, himself a lawyer, meant was that he wanted the very most lawyerly presentation, the most compelling, clearly thought-through statement of each point in the argument on both sides, from which a conclusion would emerge.

Should you do business with foreign governments that violate human rights? There's a case to be made that engagement rewards bad behavior, and another that it creates an incentive for improvement. Both have as their end point improved human rights. But isn't supporting American business an independent end worth pursuing? How important is it? Where is Arthur Liman when you need him?

When I was a law clerk, they were called "bench memos," written in advance, outlining the arguments on both sides, the strengths and weaknesses, anything we saw that the lawyers didn't.

A brilliant statement of the case doesn't eliminate the need to judge. But it allows you to see clearly what it is that you are judging, and what the choice really entails. My friends who are judges all agree that the better the lawyers, the easier it is to be a wise judge.

If it works for foreign policy and constitutional law, why not for dieting?

I quit smoking (after eight failed attempts), and it was hard. But at least when you stop smoking, you just don't do it anymore. You make one decision and you stick to it. Eating is different. You eat all the time even when you're dieting. You constantly have to make decisions, and you have to make the "right" decision over and over again, in the face of enormous temptation, or else you'll fail. It is a matter of persuasion, which is what lawyers are trying to do when they make a case. Why not make it for yourself?

If you will commit to dieting, I will give you my Miracle Diet. If you will agree to make the case for yourself before you commit bloody murder, I'll help you build a case that Johnnie Cochran couldn't touch. If you will agree to approach the task of losing weight just as you do everything else in your life that you succeed at, my diet will work miracles.

I'll start off telling you what to eat, until you decide you know better. I'll start off asking the questions, until you know better questions to ask yourself. I'll start off making the case, until you can make it for yourself.

I want to be the voice in your head when your hand reaches for the refrigerator door. I want to be there to make sure that someone is arguing against the chocolate brownie. I won't let you forget that cheating is a decision, and overeating can be slow suicide. I'll never let you off easy. My job is to engage your brain and mine on the most important decisions you will make today, and take it as seriously as it deserves, until the voice you hear inside your head is your own.

CHAPTER TWO

My Life as a Dieter

My father's mother was fat, and so were all her sisters. A "tendency," we called it. So was my mother's mother, who died when my mother was a teenager. My mother has always been thin. Not so her children.

Food was a constant issue in our family, a punishment and a reward, a source of solace and of pain. If I ever had the ability to actually feel full, I long ago lost it, in the mixed messages (eat / don't eat; clean your plate / count your calories) my family specialized in. As a kid, I would sit in the kitchen eating blueberry muffins and reading, trying to block out the noise of my mother and sister fighting. The reading was the escape. The muffins were the prison. I took a love of both, and a need for both, with me.

My mother considered it her job to watch everything we ate, to make sure we wouldn't get fat. It worked, sort of. I grew up always believing I was on the fat side, never confident that I looked just fine. Now I look at old pictures, and I don't get it. I look thin.

Watching My Weight

My mother sent me off to college with a warning: Watch your weight.

I watched my weight, just like my mother said. I watched it go up. And—without her constant attention to it—up and up. I owe a great deal to my alma mater, Wellesley, a women's college that teaches you that women can do anything. For more than twenty years, I also owed it twenty-something pounds.

Midway through freshman year, when I saw the scale touch 140 for the first time, I dropped eight pounds in four days by eating nothing but eggs and tomatoes. When the weight came back, I did it again, only to have it come back a few weeks later. By then it was Passover, and I ate nothing but matzo and jam, two pieces per meal, and the pounds went away. By summertime, they were back again.

My mother refused to send me back to college fat. I refused to be a fat sophomore. We didn't have a lot of money, but this was important to us. She took me to a diet doctor in Boston, a woman (my first woman doctor, such a role model) who gave me diet pills and put me on the following diet: Breakfast—toast, cottage cheese, six ounces of liquid. Lunch—three pieces of fruit, six ounces of liquid. Dinner—six ounces of protein, one cup of vegetables, six ounces of liquid. That's it. Simple. I remember it perfectly, even twenty-five years later, particularly the part about the water. No liquid after dinner. No cheating with ice chips, either. Insane.

I stuck to it for three weeks. I lost ten pounds. And people say overweight people have no discipline—I was working nights in a muffin shop at the time.

I went back to college literally pruned into shape, only to gain about five pounds with my first diet soda. I was so depressed I gained three more. I went to see the diet doctor, taking the subway from Wellesley myself this time, shaking with anger and desperation because I now weighed only two pounds less than I did when I first went to see her. It was all my fault, she told me. If only I'd stayed on the diet. She prescribed more pills and less water. It took me twenty years to get down to that weight again.

How's your weight? my mother would ask, in our weekly phone conversations. There, I would answer. If I wanted to be mean, I'd tell her the truth.

My last year of college, I went to Weight Watchers meetings in a church in Cambridge, where I knew no one and was the youngest by twenty years, instead of joining a group in Harvard Square where I might have found friends. Was it because I wanted to fail? Because I wanted to punish myself? Because I was trying to hide my problem? Who knows? I lasted long enough to lose ten pounds, meet a new and thoroughly inappropriate man, and start law school at the high-average end of the weight scale (naked and leaning to the right, looking toward the left) instead of the clearly overweight, which meant I hated myself the usual moderate amount.

After my first year of law school, I made the Harvard Law Review and for a time, I was the only woman among fifty men. I worked harder than any of them. And probably ate as much if not more than any of them. Friday nights, exhausted from a week of eighteen-hour days, I would head over to the TGIF in the Commons and drink too much, and then go back to work the next morning and eat too much. One of the perks at the Law Review was that there were fresh bagels and cream cheese every morning—free, even—in exchange for your seventy-hour-a-week commitment. We ordered on the basis of three per person (which totals about 750 calories, without the cream cheese, but who's counting?), but not everyone came every day, or stayed as long as I did.

My success at the Law Review, particularly after my second year, when I was elected president and appeared in *People* magazine and on *Good Morning America* and right after a stripper on local TV, was the result of a group effort mounted by my women friends. My first year of law school, I worked at Mahoney's 499 Lounge, a bar in Somerville, ten minutes and a million miles away from Harvard Law School. Once a week Suzanne would post a notice on the board: WOMEN'S CONSCIOUSNESS-RAISING GROUP, 8 P.M. (we called it that to threaten the male professors), which meant the girls would be drinking at Mahoney's that night, bucking each other up to go back to the wars. They'd hang out until I'd closed up, and then we'd go out for pancakes and eggs at one in the morning, and fall asleep in class the next day.

The group saw it as their responsibility to keep me going on the Law Review, to buck me up when a third-year student called me an "ambitious chick" (we gave him as a gift that famous poster that said "Women are not chicks") and to bring me brownies, sandwiches, lasagne, and other taste treats when the bagels ran out. Food as love, comfort, solace.

My third year, my father, who always taught me that I could do anything, died. Kate, my best friend on the Law Review, lost her husband to suicide during the same week. Seven days earlier, my sister had left an abusive marriage and had moved in with friends. My mother, who'd also gotten involved with an abusive man after my parents' marriage ended, left him the week after my father died, and she too was living with friends. My brother was a freshman at Brown. I was the president of the Harvard Law Review, with three issues left to get out, five classes I had never set foot in to pass, a prestigious clerkship lined up for September but no source of income until then, an unpaid tuition bill, a mountain of student loans, and nowhere to live once the school year ended and the dorms closed. I even had an evil stepmother, a woman to whom my father was briefly and unhappily married, whose first comment to me when I walked, shaking with terror, into the intensive care unit where the person I loved most in the world was lying near death, was: "What about the house?" They were supposed to close on a house the next day.

I called health services and told them I was having trouble sleeping, and they wisely insisted that I talk to someone as the price of a prescription for sleeping pills. I did; a warm and wise woman who told me a few useful things: that it would not be a good time for me to diet, which is what I'd planned to do during my last semester, and that I never had to talk to my stepmother again. She also taught me that it is not what happens to you in life, but how you adapt to it, that matters most. Happiness and satisfaction are choices, not simply the product of chance or fate.

Professional Gains

I waited until I got to Washington to diet, where I worked first for the law firm of Covington and Burling (which hired me after the same wise counselor advised me that I was not really in a position to worry about "selling out" right then but instead should find someone willing to hire and house me) and then for Judge J. Skelly Wright, a wonderful man, a hero of the civil rights movement, and a believer in sane working hours. I ate salads, swam at night after work, and even to my jaundiced eye looked pretty good, which didn't stop me, when I was on vacation in Florida that year with my friend Kate, from eating only eggs and cottage cheese for a week. On vacation.

The next year, I moved "up," as they say, to the Supreme Court, where I had the privilege of working for Justice John Paul Stevens. Most justices, in those days, had four or five clerks. Justice Stewart prided himself on having three. Justice Stevens decided he wanted to give it a try with two—the same number Justice Rutledge had when Stevens clerked for him. I was one of them; my co-clerk was the former president of the Stanford Law Review, Jim Liebman, who went on to become one of the nation's leading death penalty lawyers and then a distinguished professor of law at Columbia. He is a wonderful man and was the ideal partner for a year of intense work and learning, which is what we had. He also weighed less than I did.

As the year progressed, the difference in our sizes increased. We shared an office, where we could be found seven days a week. I was on a diet for the entire year. Most days, we had lunch with the justice, who still reminds me about the spinach salads I would eat every day because I was "watching myself." Gain weight, that is.

That summer, I studied for the bar and starved myself, so I would look better for my next job, working for Stephen Breyer, who was then taking over as chief counsel of the Senate Judiciary Committee, and is now on the Supreme Court himself. By the time I got there, in the summer of 1979, all of the focus was on the chairman of our committee, Senator Edward Kennedy, and the increasing likelihood that he would challenge the incumbent president, Jimmy Carter, for the Democratic nomination. The polls showed Kennedy way ahead of everyone, and the competition to be "chosen" for the campaign was considered the first step to an office in the White House. I was one of the lucky ones, and I fell in love, for a time, with presidential politics. I would put a sentence about the Equal Rights Amendment in a Kennedy speech, and two days later, the President of the United States would have a meeting with women's leaders. Cool. There is nothing like a losing campaign for those who start at the bottom, because almost everybody above you disappears. When the paychecks stop coming, most grown-ups can't afford to stay; as the prospects of victory fade, kids like me get to do more.

I got to do a lot that year. I ate pancakes in New Jersey, bagels in Florida, a million deli sandwiches in New York, pizza and Chinese food across America. I ate chicken-fried steaks in Iowa, corn dogs in Minnesota, and everything on the airplanes.

It was the first of three presidential campaigns I worked on over the next decade, all of which resulted in electoral losses for my candidates and weight gains for me. This is what you do in campaigns. You sit, you work, and you eat. There is a myth that because you're traveling all the time, living this weird life inside a cocoon from which you're supposed to know the beat of America, you never know when you'll get to eat again. The answer, of course, is always soon.

Life on the Trail

A typical campaign day involves as many as five meals and just as many snacks. You pull yourself out of bed at the crack of dawn, and wander by the staff room, where there is a full spread laid out by six A.M.—coffee, sweet rolls, danish, bagels, etc. There is usually also fruit, which takes longer to eat. You shove in the muffin, and head for the bus or the van to the first event, where there will be a holding room for the candidate, with an almost identical spread, which he won't touch, so you might as well. You then get back in the bus or van and head for the plane, where a nice hot breakfast is served en route to your next event. You land at the airport, head straight to the site for the next event, where there will be both a holding room and a staff room, both offering delicatessen sandwiches, salads full of mayonnaise, and plates of cookies and brownies. The candidate does his event, while you make phone calls and eat. Then you get back in the car or van, head back to the airport, get back on the plane, where your friends the flight attendants are getting ready to serve a nice hot lunch. And so the day goes, sometimes through three or four stops. At the airport, supporters will hand up buckets of ribs in the Midwest, pizzas in Chicago, fried chicken in the South, and you eat that too, because you're so sick of plane food, even the fancy kind. And then finally you land, and if you can keep your eyes open and aren't the one who has to stay up all night and get ready for the next day's events, you get to have fun. You go out to eat.

In real life, I taught law at Harvard, and dieted. After the 1984 campaign, I signed up with the Diet Center. The gist—you were supposed to keep a food journal and check in every day where women in white coats would weigh you and "provide support." It feels like the doctor's office, and costs a lot of money, which should be powerful incentive. But getting weighed every day is sort of stupid, since everyone's weight fluctuates, so you get depressed, and then you (if you're me) start playing little games: never drink—even a sip of water—before you weigh in; weigh in on Monday afternoon *and* on Tuesday morning and you'll show a loss. Lie. Say you had a lot of salt the night before. Did you cook your chicken on the bone? the earnest woman would ask as she pressed me to buy little packets of lemon juice to keep in my purse. No, I had my martini with an olive in it, my yogurt with fudge, my potato chips with dip. Could I trick them? Could I trick myself?

And up and down we go. Starve for the wedding, eat on the honeymoon. Everyone seems to agree that yo-yo dieting is a terrible thing, and those of us who do it would be hard-pressed to disagree. Whether or not it is physiologically more difficult to lose the same ten pounds for the fifth or sixth time, it is certainly harder on the head.

I gained the most weight during the 1988 campaign, when my responsibilities were weightiest. I was appointed campaign manager of the Dukakis for President campaign in the fall of

1987 when two close friends, John Sasso and the late, great Paul Tully, lost their jobs over an incident that by today's campaign standards would rank as a schoolyard stunt. They gave a reporter a videotape showing the similarities between a speech delivered by a British Labor candidate and one delivered by Senator Joseph Biden, then an opponent in the pre-primary days. When the story broke, the Biden people immediately "spun" it around to a question of who had leaked the tape, and everyone denied everything, including my friends. While all this was happening, I was getting ready to teach the fall semester at Harvard, having pulled back my involvement from the campaign (as it turns out at the strategic moment) because I'd decided that while it might be possible although extraordinarily difficult to teach law in Cambridge and live in California, it was absolutely impossible to work in a presidential campaign based in Boston while living the life of a newlywed in Los Angeles.

I looked pretty good on the day Governor Dukakis announced my appointment, what would turn out to be my thinnest moment of the next five years. Harvard wasn't about to let me out of my classes just because I was running a presidential campaign, so two days a week, I'd head over to Cambridge to teach. When I wasn't in class, I lived in my office, working— and ordering in food—around the clock. If that weren't enough, after twenty years as a smoker, I'd quit for the last time; it was a promise to myself and my husband that I was determined to keep. So I didn't smoke, and I ate, and we won primaries, beating Al Gore and Dick Gephardt and Bruce Babbitt and Paul Simon and the Reverend Jesse Jackson. I began the summer almost fat and happy. It was the best ride I'd ever had in politics, followed by the worst.

By mid-summer, the poll numbers were terrible, even though the horse race had us ahead of Bush. The economy was doing better, people thought the country was on the right track—all of which would help then Vice President Bush—and Dukakis was more liberal than most people realized. The worst thing anyone had to say about Bush was that he was a rich wimp, which is not as bad, politically speaking, as being considered "soft on crime." We should have been focusing on Bush, but we were stuck dealing with Jesse Jackson. We needed a peaceful convention, but we also needed to look like we were in charge. Jackson had a third of the delegates, enough to do anything he wanted other than win the nomination, and I had a stomachache that wouldn't go away.

Things got better for a while. Lloyd Bentsen was a great selection for vice-president and Ann Richards gave a great keynote. For thirty seconds, everyone thought we were geniuses. And then we came back to Boston, where we stayed for the next month, while George Bush attacked us every day. The governor was in the statehouse most of the time, or on statehouse business that he had put off for months and now could not seem to walk away from. I was in my office, eating stomach tranquilizers and getting beaten up by the press and everybody in the party because we weren't leaving Massachusetts and the White House was slipping away.

It was an ugly campaign, a watershed in presidential politics, still, for the meanness. John Sasso came back for Labor Day; I welcomed him back, wearing my friend Pam's red polka-dot suit, and managing to look half decent as I was being replaced on national television. But of course I couldn't leave; I was still the "campaign manager," he was the "vice-chair," and despite our own past friendship, there were divided loyalties, hurt feelings, and plenty of fingerpointing as things went from bad to worse. Defeat is always an orphan. Finally, my friend Chuck, who'd had a kidney transplant, took me to his doctor at Massachusetts General Hospital.

You know what they say: When the going gets tough, the tough go shopping. Filene's Basement was two buildings away from our headquarters. One particularly awful day, I found a red silk suit, size 14, in the designer corner, with a long jacket and a long skirt that hid everything better than anything else I owned, and I wore it to all the debates and big events. On election day, I rolled the waistband a few times, and went out for the last time to try to look cheerful and upbeat in interviews until the polls closed in the West.

I left Boston the Friday after the election heavier than I had ever been in my life.

I went to Rancho La Puerta, a health spa in Mexico. The place was great, but I didn't lose much weight. I tried the Diet Center again, but wiped out completely. I went to Weight Watchers for a few meetings, before deciding I hated meetings. I did battle at Jenny Craig, which tries to tell you that you have to eat beef stew on Wednesdays, and then insists on selling you the beef stew. But I don't like beef stew, I would tell my "counselor"; why can't I do two Tuesdays instead of a Wednesday, since I like Salisbury steak? Not allowed. But soon I didn't care. Three weeks into it, I discovered I was pregnant.

Epiphany at Loehmann's

I gained forty pounds during my first pregnancy, lost thirty, and then gained forty-plus back during my second. You see how the math works.

My moment of truth, diet-wise, came in the Loehmann's dressing room, a few months after my son was born. May she rest in peace, Erma Bombeck was right: There is no lesson in life that cannot be learned at Loehmann's.

What was I doing in the Loehmann's dressing room "a few months" after my son was born? I breast-fed my daughter for six months or so, until she lost interest and I lost capacity, and I'd planned to do the same with my son. But it didn't work; at the two-week visit to the pediatrician, he'd lost weight, and I was beside myself, felt guilty, a complete failure. I went to one of those medical supply places and rented a baby scale, and weighed him five or six times a day, which he fortunately does not remember, but I do. I rented a breast pump to try to give the old breasts some extra help, but it only proved how meager my supply was. He was much happier on a soy formula than he had been with me.

On the bottle, my son started gaining weight, and I started dieting. I'd diet for a week or so, then go off for a few days, then start something new. Nothing was happening. After two or three months of this, I weighed six pounds more than I did at the end of the 1988 campaign. I had plateaued at fat.

There's a lie we all like to tell about how much we weigh; and what makes it so transparently a lie is that we all use the same numbers. According to the surveys, the average American woman weighs 140 pounds and would like to weigh 125. Only the last half is true. My friend Jack taught me one of the most valuable lessons I learned in politics: never believe any number that ends in a zero or a five. Someone made it up. I said I weighed 140 for most of the time between college and Loehmann's. But the truth is, 140 was the least I weighed. I looked good at 140—it's only ten pounds more than I weigh now that I'm "thin." The problem was that I rarely weighed 140—it was more like 143, or 148, or 151 but deduct two pounds for all that salt in the popcorn, or 155, at which point I would stop weighing myself. That day in the dressing room, I had to face the fact that I was forty (well, maybe fifty) pounds plus from the weight I'd promised myself as a birthday present every year since I was eighteen.

I'd been wearing black maternity leggings nonstop for so long I was ready to burn them all. I went to Loehmann's to buy a pair of regular pants. I failed. Nothing fit. The size 10's—what I wore when I got pregnant—weren't even in the ballpark; I didn't even try, I had a closet full at home. But hope still springs eternal. I tried the size 12s. No luck. I took a deep breath. You just had a baby, I told myself. Be kind. Try on some size 14s, cheap ones, because you won't be wearing them for very long. I tried. I couldn't button them. I couldn't zip them.

Everyone knows women who were the proverbial size eight when they got married—and then they had their kids. She never lost it, we say to each other. It was the pregnancies, they always say. My neighborhood is full of Orthodox Jewish women with four children and forty extra pounds. I looked just like them, except I had two children, not four.

And that was the least of it. Being fat increases the chances that you will die young. Being a forty-year-old mother of babies makes this thought almost unbearable.

Terrible things happen to people all the time. After playing with my son at the school fair, my friends' two-year-old stopped breathing; a virus, undetectable, the autopsy said. One of my closest friends was just diagnosed with breast cancer; she joins a long list of friends and acquaintances trading notes about wig stores, chemo, and oncologists. My friend Rob's sister, a breast cancer survivor, lost her husband and two sons in a plane crash. That's just a month's worth. You get to a point in your life where you realize how fragile everything is.

Love makes the possibility of terrible things happening even more terrifying. I got married when I was thirty-three. My daughter was born when I was thirty-seven; my son, when I was forty. I love my family fiercely. Looking at my baby daughter, and three years later, my baby son, I understood the elemental power of love, how people could be moved to kill; I would kill anyone who touched them. Each night, when I would go into their rooms to listen for their breathing, as I still do, a knot of fear would grip me in my gut, the flip side of love. There is no end of things you can worry about—for them, and for yourself. I would pore over the sections of books on childhood illness, feeling my stomach turn if ever I recognized a symptom. When my doctor felt a thickening in my breast just after my daughter's first birthday, when my husband found a suspicious mole when my son was a week old, I was beside myself with fear. The high stakes of presidential politics pale before the vulnerabilities of love.

I don't swear at traffic lights. I'm nice to the dry cleaners. I don't sweat the little things. I know what matters, and how much it matters. That does not necessarily make anything easier.

This is not something my family did well. My grandfather was terrified of death, but he dealt with what he saw as his ultimate enemy the way he'd dealt with the earlier ones, in Russia and then in South America, and finally in the United States. With contempt. He smoked and drank, and nothing and no one could make him quit. Even when he was seriously ill, as he was a number of times while I was growing up, he prided himself on his stubborn refusals to follow doctors' orders. He used to steal cigarettes from my purse when I'd visit him in the hospital. He'd leave me a dollar. He made my grandmother pour schnapps into the home-squeezed orange juice and then bring thermoses to him in the hospital, right past the nurses who thought him old-fashioned for insisting on only drinking his wife's juice. He showed them. He tossed the dice, and lived to eighty-three.

My father did it the same way, but with less contempt. "My Way" was his favorite song. He smoked and drank, too, and lost the bet. It has been twenty years since he died; soon, I will have lived more of my life without him than with him. It still breaks my heart.

My mother deals with life by worrying. She worries constantly. It is her mode. If she leaves a message that doesn't begin with, "Everything's all right," I know that it isn't.

I try to deal with my fears rationally. My husband taught me how to do this. If I can teach you one thing, it is this:

You might as well assume things will turn out all right because if they do, you'll regret all the energy you wasted worrying that they wouldn't, and if they don't, your worrying obviously didn't help. So you might as well at least have enjoyed the time beforehand. You'll never look back and say, I wish I'd worried more.

I choose to be positive, to be optimistic, to remind myself that there is a very good chance that none of those terrible things will happen (*kinnehora,* as we say in Yiddish, to keep that evil eye away), that they are unusual events. It is a choice, not a natural inclination, a choice made by the lawyer in me, not by my mother's daughter.

I am an optimist, not a gambler. Optimism is not a reason for living dangerously, for not doing your part. This is the part my father never got. Blind optimism is foolhardy. But so is wasting your life worrying.

I don't know any way to approach life and remain sane and non-depressed except doing everything you possibly can to take care of yourself and your family, and then resolving to enjoy every blessed day as much as you possibly can. For me, losing weight, exercising, living differently became an act of optimism, and a kind of blessing.

My friend Copelia found me in the dressing room that day at Loehmann's; she also found me a pair of black stretch pants that were almost identical to the leggings I was ready to burn.

She tried to make me feel better, telling me it wasn't my fault. "But it is," I snapped back, which was the truth.

In the ten years we'd been friends, Copelia had seen me go on at least a dozen diets, none of them successful. "This is it," I said to her. "It's going to be different this time."

I made a decision that day that led me to where I am today. I decided that losing weight was not just important, but really important, that I had the power to do it, and that I was going to do it, once and for all. I'd been on a diet for most of my life, and now I was fat. Now or never.

I didn't get the Ten Commandments and the Books to Back It Up right there in the dressing room. That, I admit, I did myself later with the benefit of research, which some say is also how the Lord chose to accomplish it. But what I felt that day was the rush of commitment, the intensity of making a choice and binding myself to it, a covenant of my own.

Copelia and I were together a year later, when someone asked me how I'd lost all that weight. "The same way she does everything else," Copelia said, tapping her head. "She used her brain."

CHAPTER THREE

Smart Women, Stupid Diets

When I was thirteen, I would do what everybody else was doing, join what they were joining, or at least I would try. Most girls try to look exactly the same in junior high, which is why so many of us look our worst. We all wore the same color makeup, the same lipstick, the same as that model who in no other way resembled us. We ignored anyone who told us we were just throwing our money away. At forty, I was still dieting that way. Most of my friends still do. We are grown women, smart women, competent women—and we diet like teenagers. Is there a tall, blond model with a new diet? Of course it will work for me, after all, we have so much in common. Would you ask that blond model if she thought you were a good mother?

Believe Anything: The Difference Between Critical Thought and Getting Stupid

You're running a business, or the church office. Someone tells you that you can cut your phone bills in half just by using a pair of special scissors to cut the wires. Call 1-800-CUT NOW and sign up.

What do you think? You're probably a little bit skeptical. Cut the wires, and you cut your bill in half? Who are you dealing with? Do some research here. Get some references. Check it out. You'd insist on understanding how it works before you risked your phone service on it. After all, no one wants to play games with their telephone service. I mean, what if they're wrong?

In short, if someone offered to cut your phone bill in half by selling you special scissors, you wouldn't be giving your credit card number to the 800 operator quite yet. You wouldn't ignore everything you knew about fly-by-night companies because the person seemed sincere, and someone at the beauty parlor had tried it. You would research. You would analyze. You would engage in critical thought.

You're driving along flipping the dial, or clicking around the tube, and you hear something about a diet that lets you eat 5,000 calories a day, including all the cheese and butter you want, and you lose weight and never get hungry, and what do you say?

"What's the name of the book?"

My old friend Meredithe used to call it getting stupid, something we all did with men on occasion, and on diets all the time. Twenty ounces of beef in a day on the heart association diet, but no fruit for days? Sure, I'll believe it. Even if I don't, I'll try it. What have I got to lose?

I used to go the bookstore every Saturday night, looking at the diet books. Which one of you will make me thin? I would ask. I'd turn to about page 43, and start looking for chapters entitled "The Secret Fiber" to see if I could save the money and find the secret or, better yet, see through it and have a snack on the way home. When everyone did Atkins, I did Atkins. When everyone did Stillman, I did Stillman. When everyone did the Zone, I did the Zone, even though I had already lost my weight, and love carrots, which you're not allowed to eat.

Most diet books these days fit into one of two categories:

(1) big celebrities; or (2) bigger gimmicks. They have to, or they won't be published.

The problem with the big celebrities is not that their fame generally has nothing whatsoever to do with anything that would commend their views, experiences, or thoughts about dieting. I don't mind that. It's that they write their diet books after a lifetime of mostly being thin and beautiful (which is how they got to be a celebrity in the first place), during which they gained ten pounds for twenty minutes. I know what it's like, they write. Then they cut back and used low-fat yogurt and had their chefs start cooking healthy meals, and voilà. It's so easy to be thin. Most of them don't lie, but they don't have a clue. That's why Oprah is different.

The big gimmicks are much worse. There are fat-busters and carb-busters and butter-busters. Super is no longer enough; everything is mega, and meta. These days, you need a really, really big gimmick to break out if you're not a celebrity. And the beauty is they all work. For about a week. Until you revolt. And you've failed. Stick that book back on the shelf. You gain the weight back as fast as you've lost it. Faster, probably. And while it might be perfectly clear to you in any other context that your only mistake was trying to stick to it for more than a few days, you won't see it that way, I never used to.

I have nothing against gimmicks, plans, crutches, and anything else that will get you to eat less and move more. What infuriates me is when all these people whose books I have bought over the years take me for an idiot and treat me like one. Instead of explaining that their diet works because you end up eating less and moving more, they give you mumbo-jumbo that most people never read about the magical qualities of whatever gimmick they've invented. Most of us, to be honest, skip that section of the book. Wisely. But even if you read it, what you find in most of them is that the claims don't add up. I don't mean they're not true, although most scientists would say they aren't. I mean that at best, all that surplus energy-burning that you get from eating the grapefruit instead of the orange, or following the fat-buster routine, doesn't begin to equal the piece of carrot cake you'll eat in frustration. It's peanuts. No, peanuts have a lot of calories. We're talking one extra apple a day if you believe it all. At least tell us that, and give us the choice.

But the purpose of most of the books we waste our money on isn't to teach you anything. They don't want you to act like an intelligent person. They are certainly not interested in critical thought. They certainly don't say: This is novelty. That's why it works. Stick to it for a few days. Learn from that. Substitute later. They say it's rocket science, brain science, the new magic of fiber-butter-buster-mega-whatnot. We should be furious at them, but instead we end up furious at ourselves for failing at a diet that worked for all those mythical people who have spent a lifetime eating nothing but meat, fish, eggs, and cottage cheese, just like Dr. Stillman said. And I would believe it because it worked for me for five days.

You want a diet? I'll give you a diet, but I won't pretend to be God. When you're not counting, it's because I am. You can't escape the numbers.

Try Everything: Victoria and the Storefront Fen-Phen

Don't be mad at me, my friend Victoria said. I'm taking pills. She meant fen-phen.

Fen-phen, as even non-dieters surely know, is the cocktail form of two separate drugs, fenfluramine and phentermine, which were separately approved by the FDA for short-term treatment of obesity more than two decades ago. The combination was never approved, because of unknown side effects, but that didn't stop doctors from writing 18 million prescriptions for fen-phen in 1996, and 2.4 million more for the similar drug Redux, before reports of dangerous side effects led to its "voluntary" withdrawal at the FDA's insistence.

What were millions of smart women doing taking an unproven combination of drugs that would kill them? In their defense, the drug manufacturers have argued that obesity poses a bigger risk than fen-phen. But not all people taking fen-phen were clinically obese, or even close, which was one reason they were seeking medical advice at the mini-mall instead of their usual doctor's office.

In my neighborhood, I used to watch the women pull up to the clinics, well dressed, in nice cars, hardly obese. They were not the type of women who usually sought medical help next to the dry cleaner's; they would never trust their hair to a beautician they didn't know, or a colorist without references. They were particular about who did their nails at the manicure place next door. But they risked their lives to lose weight.

"My regular doctor would never give it to me," Victoria said, explaining why she got her prescription from a doctor she barely knew, in a mini-mall, instead of the doctor she would call if sickness were to strike. Of course not. She's no heavier than I used to be when I went to diet doctors and swallowed snake oil, happy that they'd give it to me, no questions asked. Who are we kidding?

I wasn't mad at my friend for taking pills. I was mad at her for getting them at the same mini-mall where she wouldn't trust the dry cleaner with her husband's shirt. I was mad at her because I like her and I don't want her to get pulmonary hypertension or heart valve disease, which would be much worse than having to give up bagels and walk more, which—if she did—would take the weight off. I was mad at her for being stupid about her life, when she's smart about everything else.

Rank the following in the order in which you provide the most care.

Your car	Your shoes
Your dog	Your garden
Your children	Your houseplants
Your lover	Your fish
Other loved ones	Your body

You know how to score it.

Set Yourself Up for Failure:
Too Busy to Diet, but Not to Care

It doesn't necessarily take time to lose weight—you can buy packaged food, eat fruit, get a salad at McDonald's—but it does take energy. For most of us, the busier we are, the more we eat, the less we exercise, the more we gain. I look at my dieting history, and the moral is pretty clear. The harder I worked, the fatter I got.

I used to joke with my friends, at the end of eighteen-hour days, that someone should have told us that this is what the feminist revolution would bring. Women are busier than ever before; most effectively work at least two jobs, and with aging parents, it can easily be three. What makes it harder is that most families are no more work-friendly than workplaces are family-friendly. Families like the introduction of work into their lives no more than the other way around. They have very strong views on things like sitting down at the computer after dinner to work, or working on weekends, and besides, who wants to miss all the good stuff? So you're stretched and you're pulled and you're working hard. You put yourself last and at the end of the day, woe is you, no time for dieting, no time for exercise, no time to take care of yourself. You eat what's on the plate, grab what's at hand, and gain weight. Sound familiar?

There are two logical approaches you can take if you're busy, and you want to lose weight.

1. You can decide that losing weight is important, and make space in your life for it.

2. You can decide that losing weight is not so important, and not make a place for it.

There's only one approach you could take that would be really stupid:

3. You can decide that losing weight is really important, that you really care intensely about how much you weigh, but that you're not going to treat it as a priority in your life. You'll act as if it weren't important, even though you deeply believe otherwise.

Shortly before the Democratic Convention in 1988, I looked at myself in the mirror and decided that I was about to embark on an amazing journey—first woman presidential campaign manager takes over faltering effort and wins nomination. And for my moment in the sun, I would be . . . size 14, give or take. I signed up for Diet Center, which was an idiotic idea, requiring me to add one more "meeting" a day and a rigid diet to an inflexible, unbelievable, and utterly inhuman schedule. I was going to fail. I was wasting my money. I was lying to myself. And this is when I was supposed to be a genius.

My friend Martha just started a new job. She's working all the time. She grabs food. She has no time for dieting. Besides, it's boring compared to her exciting job.

But she makes time every day to weigh herself. She's joined an expensive gym she doesn't go to. She wears tailored clothes that get uncomfortable at the first sign of tightness, which is supposed to keep her thin but instead makes her miserable.

She could cut back a little, get a trainer to come to her office or her house early in the morning (she could afford it), get meals delivered (that too), and she'd lose weight. Too extravagant.

Or she could get her suits let out a little, or get some elastic put in around the sides, and decide that this year is for work. Not a chance. It matters too much to her. Besides, she's convinced that when she looks good and feels confident, she's better at her job, and she's probably right.

So here's what this (otherwise) smart and successful woman is doing instead. She doesn't go to the gym, doesn't have the trainer come in, doesn't even take time for a walk. She doesn't have her suits altered. She weighs herself every morning and beats herself up for being fat. It makes her so miserable that she just . . . eats more. She skips breakfast, snacks too much, rolls up her skirt, and keeps an eye out for any miracle diets that might cross her desk. She's still waiting, and in the meantime, she's gaining a pound or two a week—just about what she was losing last year at this time. She hates herself for it, but feels powerless to stop. Hundreds of people work for her.

Martha knows she is being stupid, at least when she stops to think about it, which she therefore studiously tries to avoid. But she has a ready excuse for that as well; defense lawyers have nothing on chronic dieters when it comes to excuses. She is not being stupid. She is being selfless. She is taking care of everyone's needs before her own. What a wonderful woman she is. Everyone loves Martha. A smart, successful woman who can singlehandedly turn herself into everyone's victim.

Ouch.

I told you I wouldn't let you off easy.

It is Mother's Day, and I'm on the radio. Doug is my first caller. "What made Mom special," he tells us, "is that she always put herself last. If there wasn't enough ice cream to go around, she'd go without. If there wasn't enough for everyone to have seconds, she'd give you hers. And she never complained. It made her happy."

"Your mother was a saint," I tell Doug. What else can I say?

No one ever says they loved their father because he always put himself last. Since when is putting yourself last a measure of love? For most of us, it's not the road to sainthood, it's the route to the refrigerator, self-hatred, and a less successful life.

If you lose weight and get in shape, the chances are that you will live a longer and healthier life. You will cut your risk of cancer, heart disease, diabetes, and stroke. You will be more active and spend less time in the hospital. You will be less of a burden to others. You are more likely to be there when they need you. You will look better in clothes. You will look better out of clothes. You will have more sex. You will like yourself more. You will have healthier pregnancies. You will do better at work. You will be able to walk up steps without getting winded. You will be able to buy cheaper clothes. You will be kinder to animals. You will like yourself better.

When I was growing up and we'd go to fancy restaurants for special occasions, my mother would never order a meal for herself. Instead, she'd eat from everyone else's plate. The consequences of her martyrdom were that the rest of us got less of the special dinner. She wasn't giving, she was taking. Sorry, Mom, but it's true. Sometimes what we like to think of as selfless is anything but.

If you always put yourself last, then the busier you get, the further back in line you'll be. The same priorities that used to leave a little more time for you will now leave you with less than none. When this happens, most of us do not feel like Mother Teresa, even if that is what others choose to believe of us. We feel like grouchy, miserable martyrs. It's enough to make you eat two pieces of pie instead of one, at least the next chance you get. Sorry, Doug.

Martyrdom at the expense of your health, happiness, and well-being is stupid and self-defeating. It is not a gift to your family; your good health would be. No one will thank you for it. No one should. Taking bad care of yourself is not a favor to anybody. It is stupid, and you are smart.

Besides, it's not even honest.

If I told you that I had a secret—a genuine, guaranteed, secret way to lose weight and look great, but you'd have to go get a special potion four times a week, an hour door to door (that's four hours a week) and I promised miraculous results, would you do it? No matter what it cost? No matter what time the appointment was? The answer is yes, right? So enough with the martyrdom.

CHAPTER FOUR

What It Takes

You open one eye. Your husband, if you have one, is out of town, your children, if you have them, are screaming for some reason, the toilet is overflowing, the disposal broke last night, your best friend is having a biopsy, and you have deadlines at work. Good morning.

What do you do?

Of course you don't panic. It's only Tuesday. What do you do? You do what you do every day.

You assume a positive stance: Your husband is working, thank God. Your kids are breathing, or they couldn't be screaming. How lucky that there will be two things for the plumber to fix today to justify the minimum charge. There's nothing going on today that you can't handle. In other words, up and at 'em—you can do it.

Note what you don't do: This is not a great time to curse your husband for being out of town or for not existing. It is not a good time to blame the sexist schools for not teaching girls shop, so we could fix the toilets and disposals ourselves. It will not move you forward. Who's got time for it?

Second, take charge. Come up with a plan. Decide how you're going to do it. Set priorities. How many toilets do you have? Is there at least one available? Make your goals realistic.

This is not the morning to reorganize your closet or pay bills. Plan ahead. Arrange for the kids to go to the neighbors' after school.

Note what you don't do: You don't call your sister/mother/ whomever to get her permission to skip the breakfast dishes. Your own mother might do it differently; mine, for instance, would always make the bed first, even before getting dressed. You don't go looking for a book that will tell you what the magic ingredient is that means your kids will never cry. Kids cry.

You do what has to be done. You turn off the toilet, call the plumber, get dressed, make school lunches, get the kids to school, send the file on e-mail, let the plumber in, pick up your friend, check in at work, and then while she's in the doctor's of-fice, you can go downstairs and get one of those delicious mocha things with a nice blueberry muffin . . .

STOP.

This is a terrible plan for the day.

Well, I'm sorry, it's not such a great day ahead . . . and if a blueberry muffin and a mocha thing help me get through the ex-perience . . .

Eight hundred calories. You'll consume eight hundred calo-ries. In how long?

What?

How long will it take you to eat eight hundred calories? Would you give the muffin five minutes? Maybe six?

But it's my only pleasure . . .

A pleasure? You call it a pleasure to eat a muffin on the ele-vator at the hospital, while you're waiting for a friend to have a biopsy? And then your pants will be tight, and you'll feel unbe-lievably tired in about half an hour, after the sugar high is over, and that muffin is sitting in your stomach, waiting to push the scale up tomorrow, which of course will leave you feeling guilty and disgusted with yourself, which will in turn lead you to take the kids to McDonald's instead of the soup place where you'd all eat healthier, which is what a good mother would do, by the way, but you must not be thinking of that or you wouldn't be coating your arteries with fat and grease when heart disease is killing more women each year . . . Maybe you'll be next for the biopsy. Go take a walk. Look in some store windows. Cruise the bookstore.

Note: I will do anything to win, including playing the bad mother card to the hilt. Go to a therapist to get rid of your guilt; me, I'm just going to use it against you.

Tales from the Front:
The Producer Who Was Afraid to Ask Questions

Producers tell people what to do. That is their job. Mary works in Hollywood, at one of the networks, and this morning, I am hanging around because the people in New York told me to come at the wrong time. They also have the feed going back at the wrong time, and three other things are screwed up. In the middle of all this chaos, Mary is perusing the daily commissary menu. She is too busy to pack a lunch, too busy to diet, too busy to cook. Her sister has been living with her, making wonderful dinners to make up for the fact that she's overstayed her welcome. Mary is getting fat.

She tells Doris and me that she's been gaining weight steadily since her sister moved in, as she circles number three. Doris and I peer over her shoulder. Number 3: Chicken with vegetables and rice.

"Get the sauce on the side," Doris (who's just lost fifteen pounds) says.

"And ask them to steam it," I add.

She looks at us like we're crazy. Ask for the sauce on the side? Ask for them to steam it? She wouldn't dream of making such extraordinary requests of the lunchroom. I'm sure they wouldn't do special orders, she tells me. But, of course, she's never asked. She's busy.

She gets back on the other line and tells New York that they now have ninety seconds to get the feed turned around so that the L.A. guest can see New York, and next time, could they please take a little more care with the guest's time . . .

"So why don't you ask your sister to stop cooking for you?" I ask.

"Because what she really needs to do is ask her to move out," Doris chimes in.

But Mary can't do that. She can't ask her sister to move out. There's a long story about her mother, and you don't want to hear . . .

"Just ask her to cook low-fat," I say. "Buy her a cookbook, and tell her it would really help you, and she'll be grateful."

The guest complains; they still haven't got the feed right. Mary picks the phone back up, and makes clear just what she needs and when she needs it. In no uncertain terms. To New York, not the lunchroom.

The First Step: Always Take Responsibility

You can do almost anything if you take responsibility. And you can do almost nothing if you don't.

The first step to success in any business project is always to take responsibility. You can't move forward if you're looking backward, figuring out what went wrong and whose fault it is. If you spend all your time reliving the reasons you got fired, and why your old boss was wrong, you'll never find a new job. Don't give me excuses, we say to our children all the time.

It's not fair that you're overweight. It's not fair the way the world treats overweight people. The world discriminates against overweight people. Less research is done than the numbers and needs warrant, because thin people mistakenly assume that it's a level playing field, that overweight people are fatter because they're less disciplined. Ascribing fault to overweight people for their condition makes it easier for the rest of society to do less to prevent and treat obesity. It's the same argument you hear from people who say society should spend less on AIDS since those who are sick are increasingly those who have engaged in high-risk conduct. But it's never applied to lung cancer.

It also turns out to be wrong. We are not all created equal. We are only lately coming to understand more about what makes some people eat more and others less, some want more, some burn calories more efficiently. Change the chemistry of the brain, and you change what people actually want to eat. Imagine being born that way. Some people are.

It's not my fault, I used to argue, first against my mother, later against myself. I can't help that I want more to eat, that candy tastes better than apples, that Nana was fat and so were all her sisters.

We spend much of our time these days in what passes for public discourse debating whose fault everything is, and who should be blamed. It's the ultimate triumph of negativity. Instead of asking who should solve the problem, we debate who caused it. We succeed not by change, but by finding the right person to blame.

Why apply those tactics to ourselves?

It's not your fault that you were born with a slow metabolism, an inactive thyroid, or less serotonin circulating in your brain. It's not your fault that you were raised by the parents who raised you in the culture you lived in. But you're still responsible for how you look, how you feel, being your best.

We expect disadvantaged kids to obey the law, even if it's harder for them; welfare mothers to find work, even if it's harder for them. It's hard for you to lose weight. For me too. It's even harder for my sister. But we can still do it. It's just harder. No one is force-feeding us, are they? Even if they put the food in front of you, they can't make you eat it. Other people can make it harder, for sure, and we all need strategies for dealing with that. But no one can make it impossible.

You can't make yourself smarter, taller, or younger, no matter what you do. You can't do anything about the gene pool you're composed of. But you can make yourself look better and feel better and live longer by getting in shape. Compared to changing your genes, it's rather easy. You eat better, you exercise, and it happens. You don't need to be rich. You don't need to go into the hospital for a face-lift. This will make a much bigger difference. You can make yourself look better all by yourself. It's not like winning the lottery. It doesn't require luck. It doesn't even require much skill. Exercise is just as good for you if you're uncoordinated.

You are not fat because you have a hard life. You are not fat because you have a slow metabolism. You are not fat because you are poor, harried, hurt, lonely, overworked, stressed out, depressed, or disabled. You may have been victimized, but you're not doomed to be a victim. You are fat because you don't eat right, and don't exercise enough, for you.

We are dealt the hand we are dealt, but it is the genius of the human spirit that turns that into a starting point. What you do with that hand is your responsibility, and your choice.

So stop blaming your mother. Stop blaming your genes and

your job. Stop looking for someone else to take responsibility. Stop blaming the magazines and the male culture for celebrating slim women. Stop blaming the work and the kids for leaving you too exhausted to diet; women who have both work and family happen to be happier, according to the studies, and most women want both, so if you, like me, are one of those lucky enough to be blessed with a family and steady work, don't complain. We're lucky. Consider it a blessing and a challenge.

For years, I told myself that my problem was that I just didn't have enough discipline to lose weight. But that's ridiculous. Whatever my many weaknesses, no one who has ever met me would say that I lacked discipline. I've been working since I was fifteen years old. I've worked hundred-hour weeks when I could barely see straight, dragging myself out of bed in the dark, working shit jobs and putting up with horrendous abuse. Things that are *really* important we do no matter how hard they are. We work when we'd like to play, get up when we'd like to sleep, care for our kids no matter how much we're privately hurting. We do what we have to do.

Things that are just important, as opposed to really important, go right by the boards. I would like to be neater. I'm sort of a slob. My desk is always a mess. I search for shoes and socks. I never know where my keys are. It would be much better, for everybody in my family, if I were more organized. But I never will be. Because given a choice between organizing my desk and playing with my kids or reading a good book or even trying to write one, I will never clean my desk. It's a choice, at its core, and in making it I reveal what I really believe: being organized really isn't that important to me. It's very hard to do things which aren't really important to you when there's lots of reasons pushing in the other direction. Is dieting really important, or isn't it? If it is, then you will do what it takes to succeed. If it isn't, then up against all other commitments we have, a diet doesn't stand a chance.

Friends of ours have a child who began having seizures as a baby, which could not be controlled with medication, and were steadily increasing in severity and duration until they discovered a special ketogenic diet program that had been developed at Johns Hopkins University and has controlled the seizures. The parents have devoted their energies to supporting research and publicizing the diet to other parents. They hardly consider it a burden. A gift. So easy. And it saves his life.

If someone told you your child needed one special meal every day, or twenty minutes of physical therapy, and he or she could be good as new, would you resent the severe intrusion on your time, or be grateful that it was so easy?

If you don't have a child, ask the same question about your pet. Still true. About your mom, your best friend, a friend's child. Still true. Who wouldn't you begrudge a mere twenty minutes, a frying pan, an extra bag of carrots at the market? Is that really so much?

You have a new project. It's called getting yourself in shape. It is every bit as important as the running toilet, your kids' lunches, and the memo that was due two days ago.

What it takes to diet successfully is what it takes to do everything else you're going to do today: focus and energy, determination, some common sense; a positive attitude; organization; flexibility and tenacity; a willingness to forgive. It's all the familiar stuff. What's unfamiliar is its object. You.

CHAPTER FIVE

Making the Case for Yourself

It is perverse. There is no other word for it. We want to lose weight, we know how to lose weight, we know it's important to lose weight, we beat ourselves up if we don't lose weight, we have the power to lose weight, we will spend money we don't have to lose weight, and we still fail. It should be enough, all that: enough evidence, enough motivation, enough reward, and certainly enough money. Is there any doubt in your mind that you want to be thin? We risk our lives to be thin.

And then we eat a 600-calorie blueberry muffin on the elevator, two 300-calorie bagels on the car ride home, a piece of pizza and a hot dog while we're sitting in the stands, two donuts in the buffet line.

And they sit in our stomach, making us fat and making our pants tight, and we hate ourselves and feel guilty . . .

Why? Why do we do it?

It is not logic. Logic would tell us that no matter how lousy a day it is, an 800-calorie snack will only make it worse. Experience tells us that. But who thinks about that when you're about to eat a blueberry muffin?

If you stopped to think about it, you probably wouldn't do it.

Ultimately, you will need your head to set the rules of your own diet, after the Miracle. Indeed, the purpose of Susan's Miracle Diet—its miraculous structure, if you will—is to train your brain to make the decisions I'll be making for you at the outset.

You also use your head to plan ahead and avoid disaster. You use your head to come up with lies, explanations, or excuses to give you the time in the day to exercise, make a fruit salad, go to Weight Watchers.

But the most important way you use your head is to constantly convince your belly, your sweet tooth, your inner child, and everybody else that's hankering for a donut / muffin / hot dog / double bagel en auto that you are on the Miracle Diet and you don't really want that glob of cholesterol, fat, and sugar masquerading as a taste treat, that you want to be thin, look great, live long, stay healthy, and maybe even turn a few heads along the way. You use your head to make the case. You use your head to lay bare the devil in the donut, in the hope that most of the time, once you do, you'll eat an apple instead.

How I Learned to Go Out on Saturday Night and Not Be Afraid of Earthquakes

I am afraid of earthquakes, which is certainly rational and reasonable, since I live in an old house in Los Angeles.

After my children were born, I didn't want to leave them on Saturday night, or ever take a trip, because I worried that there would be an earthquake. This is no way to live.

So every time my husband and I would go out, I would make him explain to me, in somewhat excruciating detail, how it was that the chance of an earthquake that night was extremely, extremely small, and that we had taken all the appropriate precautions, and that having a social life, the two of us, was important to our marriage (my parents never went away and they got divorced; this one I would do myself, to great effect, in my head, while my husband reaffirmed the handy locale of our wrench).

In other words, with some help from me, he would make the case for going out, for not being paralyzed by fear, which even I'm smart enough to recognize is, as a matter of logic, pretty persuasive. And we'd go out, and I'd feel better.

After a while, he—or I—could make the case in shorthand. These days, I don't even make it; I acknowledge it sometimes, wave in its direction, bring it back out after an aftershock, hold on to it once in a while when the movie theater rumbles. But most of the time, I'm hardly conscious of it. I'm persuaded.

Most of the time, I forget to worry, which must mean I'm not worried.

Most of the time, I don't even look at the donuts on the buffet table, which must mean I don't want them.

Why I Don't Want Donuts

Of course I don't want donuts. I'm on a diet. At this moment in time, when the closest donut shop is a mile away, I can tell you at great length and in some detail why it is I don't want donuts, and the case is overwhelming. Even stronger than the case for going out on Saturday night. Which is why this is such a good time to prepare for the battles of the future.

A lawyer is an advocate, and a case is an exercise of advocacy. Its purpose is not to dazzle or delight; it doesn't have to be the most fun to watch or the most interesting to listen to. It has only one object. To win. To persuade.

How a lawyer presents that case will vary tremendously depending upon whom she is trying to persuade, and in what context. In the appellate court, the lawyer might get ten minutes of silence to state her case, and then not get in a word edgewise for the remainder of the time. You have to walk in knowing the two or three points you need to hammer home, you need to see quickly any vulnerabilities and plug them, and you need to play to the judges you're facing. And you generally have to do it in full sentences. An argument to the jury is a totally different matter, even if it's on the same case. It will focus on different issues, take a different tone, push different buttons. Jury arguments aren't meant to be read; they are meant to be heard, a different medium entirely, and they are intended for the twelve people sitting there, not for the lawyer's review.

In the case of dieting, making the case is both easier and harder. It's easier because the audience is always the same person—you—and you never have to use full sentences. But one person can take many different forms, not all of them logical or rational. And decisions and temptations are everywhere: you're on call every waking hour, if she stops long enough to call you, that is.

You're ready to go on a diet. You're ready to lose the weight this time. Right? That's what you told yourself when you bought this book, what you've been telling yourself, I hope, as you've been reading along. You are *ready*.

So tell me why. Take out a piece of paper, and make a list of the reasons. Do it in shorthand. Do them as pictures. Construct the case. Why do you want to lose weight?

Why do you want to lose weight enough to look the devil in the eye and tell him to keep his donuts?

Why should you be able to win any fight if you can remember to pick the fight in the first place? What's your case?

This is what you're going to need to remember, what you're going to invoke, in one form or another, about a million times in the days ahead . . . if you can remember to remember.

My Case for Losing Weight
by Susan Estrich

1. Vanity. As in, "Well, that's what you say now, but it's not what you're going to say when your clothes are tight on Saturday night."

You know that losing weight and getting in shape are about the most important things you can do to live a long and healthy life, which is the greatest gift you can give to yourself and to the people you love. That should be enough. But for most of us, at least some of the time, it isn't, and telling yourself that it "should be" doesn't make it so. So what can you do? Embrace vanity.

The number-one reason women give for wanting to lose weight is to look better. You may be embarrassed to say it out loud, but you're certainly not alone. The challenge is not to put vanity in its place, but to make sure it carries its weight. I'm all for vanity: it's the only hope against the cheeseburger.

Feeling good about how you look is incredibly important to how well you do. We all know that. If you walk into a room feeling like you look terrific, things will go better, whether it's a business meeting or a high school reunion. That reality is only oppressive when you feel lousy about yourself. It's a source of tremendous power, not to mention fun, when you feel good. Vanity can save your life, if you embrace it in a healthy way. More on this later.

2. Guilt. (Sorry, I told you I didn't solve all my problems.)

As in, "You have two young children, how can you not take care of yourself? How can you increase the chance that you won't be here when they need you?"

3. Fear. As in, "Remember how awful you looked that day in the Loehmann's dressing room when the size 14 pants wouldn't fit?" Fat and forty, what fun. Did you know that most married men who have affairs have their first one within a year of the birth of their second child? One of those useful tidbits a friend passed on right about that time.

4. The picture of myself that I carry around in my head, in a size 6 sparkly slip dress at the White House, dancing with the president, one year later.

5. The memory of my father, who didn't take care of himself, and never saw his grandchildren; the thought of Uncle Joe and Aunt Ceil, who are traveling in their eighties, not sitting in an apartment nursing their tired bodies.

6. Whoever among my friends and acquaintances was diagnosed most recently with breast cancer or colon cancer, and me not doing my best to live a long and healthy life.

7. The next major social event on my schedule.

8. The next major work event on my schedule.

9. Clothes—what I have, what I want, what I can't afford to replace if I gain weight.

10. The fact that you can't go on a book tour for a diet book if you gain all the weight back . . .

Make your own list—words, pictures, symbols. You're the only one who needs to understand it. It's all the things that matter more than the buttery taste and full belly you get from whatever it is that you're not going to eat. It's the crib sheet for your argument. It belongs on the refrigerator, or on the kitchen door, or in the middle drawer of your desk, or maybe all of the above. Wherever you hang it, it belongs first and foremost in a prominent place in the gray matter, to be used as needed, until you don't even realize that's what you're doing. Brainwashing, they call it, when it's the enemy's agenda. I prefer to think of it as reeducation. If you don't want to tell people you're on a diet, tell them your brain is in training.

Mens Rea

All the lists in the world don't help you if you don't consult them at the right moment. The critical thing isn't what's going on in your head now, but what's happening inside it in the buffet line. The answer is: Probably nothing. That's how you're going to get away with it. Without even going to law school, you've already got your defense ready. You lack a guilty mind.

There is a traditional common law rule that says that in order to commit a crime, you have to do a voluntary act with a bad intent. If the police drag you out of your house, you're not guilty of public drunkenness. It's not your fault; and besides, you didn't do anything wrong. It seems clear enough, until you hear the sad tale of someone like Mr. Decina, a squib in the casebook that sheds light on some of the hardest problems in the law, at least as they relate to dieting.

Mr. Decina fell into a state of unconsciousness while driving his car, hitting and killing a pedestrian. He is sorry. But his lawyer will surely argue that you can't charge an unconscious man with homicide, any more than you can charge the drunk dragged onto the street with public drunkenness.

Right?

Not so fast. Why was Mr. Decina unconscious?

Because he was having an epileptic seizure.

Does that help? Yes, but not enough. What else do you need to know?

Was it his first?

At the moment of impact, the first epileptic seizure will look like the third or the tenth. But the man who sets out to drive not knowing he has epilepsy has done something different—albeit at an earlier moment than the one we first focused on—than the man who gets in the car aware that he faces a higher risk of a seizure than the rest of us.

Did Mr. Decina know he was going to have a seizure when he left his house this morning? If someone had said to him, You will have a seizure and kill someone at the corner, would he have gone out this morning?

No. He's not a hit man. He's not an intentional killer. His purpose is not to kill someone, even if that's what he's about to do.

So what is he thinking when he gets in the car?

It's a mens rea question. We're examining just how guilty his mind is. That's the primary way we draw lines among people who have done the same thing. A hired hit man who runs down his victim for money is guilty of premeditated and deliberate murder, for which the penalty may be death. Mr. Decina, according to classical theory, is at most reckless, if he knew he was taking a substantial risk when he set out to drive, and did it anyway; if he didn't even realize he was taking a risk, if he didn't even think about it when he got in the car, then he is merely negligent, a state of mind that criminal law usually doesn't even bother to punish.

In each case, of course, the victim is equally dead, and the driver is the direct cause of it. What varies is the intent of the driver in striking the pedestrian: How purposeful was he? The worst killer is the premeditated killer, the killer who plans it out, has a motive for doing it, actually decides to break the law and then breaks it. It's one thing to drive too fast, take your eyes off the road, drive with an impairment, even; we can identify, or at least empathize, with those drivers, to some extent, and their liability varies accordingly. But to set about to kill someone—to run them down in cold blood—is as bad as you can be.

What's the rule? The less attention you pay to doing something, the less blameworthy you are. Intention is a measure of fault. It's not murder if you aren't paying attention. It's a lesser crime, or maybe none at all. Sound familiar?

This is exactly how most of us eat. It makes perfect sense. It will also make you fat. Calories don't count so much when you're standing up in front of the refrigerator, or eating off somebody else's plate, because you don't really mean to be eating them. We eat things on the fly that we would never sit down and order. It's easier.

It is not, unfortunately, how the body works. Eating donuts is a strict liability offense, from your body's point of view. They're just as fattening when you shovel them in out of the bag as if you sat down and ate them one bite at a time. You don't get less fat if you eat standing up, on the fly, without premeditation and deliberation. In fact, it's quite the opposite. What you accomplish by doing it on the sly, with less attention focused, is to eat more of the things you would never touch if you were treating it as a decision. Most of us who have weight problems have them not because of our premeditated and deliberate eating, but because of what we eat recklessly and negligently, without even giving the other side a chance to make the case.

The Elusive Promise of Mindful Eating

So all you have to do is take a deep breath and pay attention, right? Wrong. Wishful thinking.

Eating is not supposed to be good or bad, the experts tell us, it's just eating. The way you're supposed to lose weight is not by going on a diet but by embracing a new lifestyle in which you stop seeing food as an enemy, listen to your body, feed it what it wants, and you live happily ever after.

What a wonderful thought. No rules. No pain. All you need to do is tune in and you'll get a symphony. All you need to do is pay attention to what you're eating, and you'll eat salad. Magic.

I have been to a number of nutrition workshops which were really quite wonderful, led by lovely people who encouraged us to accept and love our bodies, to heed their wishes, to resolve to do nothing more than eat slowly, putting the fork down between every bite, chewing deliberately, eating when you're eating, thinking when you're thinking.

I try to do it. I remind myself to put my fork down between bites, not to take the next bite until I'm finished chewing. Taste the food. Sounds simple. It is simple. Look around a restaurant and no one is doing it. Now if it's so simple, and if it's all you have to do to eat less, why isn't everyone doing it? Why wasn't I?

This is the idea behind a food journal. Writing something down forces you to be aware that you're doing it. Since most of us do most everything, especially overeating, with as little consciousness as possible, increasing the attention you pay to it will likely be either revealing—Do I really eat so much in a day? you're supposed to ask yourself, as if you really don't know— or, more likely, its own restraint. You won't want to write down two potato chips, so you won't eat them. Forced to confront what you're doing, you don't do it. Mr. Decina might well have gone back in the house if someone had just followed him outside and underlined for him what he was about to do.

Food journals never worked for me. I just lied. When I remembered. Which frankly, wasn't all that often. How many carrots did I have? Who knows? Who cares? In my case, if I'm eating carrots, not carrot cake, I'm fine.

I meditate. I practice breathing. I'm open to reincarnation. I've been to healers. I have a favorite psychic. I'm ready to believe. But I have bad news for you. If I depended on mindfulness to get me thin or keep me there, I'd be fat. I'm sorry to say that but it's true. I wish I could tell you that you could breathe your way to beauty, but why in the world would you believe me if I did? Why would a majority of Americans be overweight if you could?

The normal state of eating is to shovel in food unconsciously. As wonderful as it is to pay attention to each mouthful, I don't know anyone outside of professional nutritionists who does this with any regularity. Look around at the mall, or at the fanciest restaurant you know. You'll see the same thing. Everyone shovels in their food. Most of the time, we eat like we're driving at the same time, whether we are or not. Even thin people do this. Everyone does this. It may well be harder to change than losing weight.

What's worse, human nature being what it is, under a general edict to eat mindfully all the time, the time you're likely to pay least attention is when you need to most. Sure, you'll eat mindfully when you're enjoying your morning melon. We'll munch the grapefruit slowly. Not the treat.

When a donut speaks to you in a buffet line, you will not premeditate and deliberate. If you're going to eat it, you're going to grab it and eat it fast, before anyone has a chance to notice, particularly you. You are not going to make an announcement, hold a meeting, take a vote. If you stop to think about it, you'll order oatmeal. In every survey of women's eating habits that I've seen, the pattern of secret eating stands out. No one eats mindfully standing in front of the refrigerator. No one eats mindfully from the container. No one mindfully eats three donuts from a paper bag on the bus, train, car. The five minutes you fail to eat mindfully in the day will be the five minutes when you're eating the bad stuff, and undermining everything else you've done all day.

Imposing a Duty of Care

This is not a problem unique to dieting. Mr. Decina is a law-abiding citizen, not a hit man on the loose. So are most drunk drivers. But at the moment they get in the car, they don't think: "I'm taking a foolish risk that could result in serious injury to myself and other people." No, they lie to themselves, they kid themselves, they tell themselves stories that wouldn't last thirty seconds on cross: "I'm late, I'm fine, I'll be extra careful. . . ." If they think at all.

Dieters do exactly the same thing. "I'll only have one bite, I'll make up for it later, I'll stop if it's not good. . . ." If we say anything at all.

And while it's all well and good to say that in the eyes of the Lord and the theorists, you're less blameworthy when you act this way, you're just as fat, and your victims are just as dead, and when you count up the numbers, drunk drivers kill a lot more people than hit men.

The prospect of punishment if they should lose control and kill someone doesn't stop drunk drivers, it didn't stop Mr. Decina, and it doesn't stop most dieters. It's too easy to lie to yourself when the devil has you by the short hairs. "Just a bite of each. I'm on a diet," we say perkily, as we pile a donut, a danish, and a muffin next to the fruit on the plate that will never be touched. Mostly we don't say anything at all. We're not thinking, remember. We're heading for a taste treat. Mr. Decina is late, has a hot date, an important meeting. And in his case, it is statistically right that the chances of an accident are slim, but we still don't want him driving, and neither would he, if he were thinking about it rationally. It's a pointless risk, like you and that stale donut that's staring you down, and will lead directly to muffins, which leads to pizza for lunch, in the version of the domino theory that always turns out to be right.

So how do we stop the drunk driver? How do we stop Mr. Decina? Most important, how do you stop yourself? We're not just in the business of punishing people after the fact; we want to prevent crime and save lives, not just lock people up; we especially want to lose weight. But it's damn difficult to deter the drunk or disabled driver with the prospect of something he doesn't think is going to happen, happening.

How do we turn an act of reckless disregard into an act of intentional wrongdoing (which you of course would never do)? Very simple. We impose a duty of care. We make a rule. We set the speed limit at sixty, instead of just punishing people who cause accidents by driving too fast. Ignorance is no defense. Neither is a broken speedometer, which should lead you to get yours fixed. We punish drunk drivers if we catch them, not if they kill someone.

The most common explanation for why every society needs rules is that it allows us to live together in a civilized way, which is obviously true. But rules don't just protect us against each other's wrongs. They also protect us from ourselves.

We're deciding now, when we're thinking rationally, instead of later, when we've had a few, when we're in a hurry, late for an appointment, facing a donut shop.

The most important rule for summiting Everest and not dying is the turn-around time. By the time you get that high, there is an excellent chance that you will be unable to think straight, quite literally, suffering from hypoxia. So guides impose a flat rule that if you are not at the summit by two P.M. you must turn around. When two P.M. comes, after years of effort, and weeks of brutal sacrifice, you will not want to turn around, and you will "think" that it's safe to proceed. But your thinking will be impaired. That is why you can't trust it, why the rule must be followed without question. Rob Hall, who led climbers up Everest in the spring of 1996, was quoted as saying, "I can't trust myself to turn around at the right time, and I'm a guide. So I'm going to promise myself, and everyone else, that come two o'clock, we turn around, no matter what. Your brain is going to stop working at two o'clock." A few days later, apparently at the urging of his clients, Hall ignored the turn-around time, and he and some of the clients perished.

Even when your brain is certifiably nonfunctional, a rule will sound an alarm when you're about to cross it. Two o'clock. Turn-around time. Donuts. No donuts. It is very difficult to reach mindlessly for a donut when you know you don't eat donuts. Before your fingers touch the donut, you think a donut—no donuts. A donut. You have a rule against donuts. "It would be wrong." The members of the team who turned back survived.

In a nonhypoxic state, a rule can do even more: it provides the occasion for you actually to let Johnnie or Marcia or Alan make that case. Once you've remembered to remember, if that's not enough, they'll make the pitch, exposing the donut's slimy underside and how it will look on your hips. Donuts. No donuts. Early death. Ugly thighs. Bad mother.

But perhaps the most important function that rules serve is to force the rulemaker to look ahead, to go beyond the questions of immediate gratification and basic survival to plan for her future and make decisions about how she—or we—intends to live. We commit to allowing our better instincts to govern our rasher ones.

Decisions you make in advance about what you are and

aren't going to eat will be different than what you would likely do if you were just trying to do your best in the face of temptation; the shopping list that you make at home is always different than what you end up buying when you're hungry. The diet you decide on in advance will be smarter and healthier than the one you make up as the day goes along. Johnnie will at least get a chance to argue, and he'll remind you of what happened to Mr. Decina.

You can't convict Mr. Decina of homicide, his lawyer argued at the time. You're punishing him for what happened while he was unconscious. It's no different than if he'd had a heart attack.

The court didn't buy it. He wasn't unconscious when he got in the car, they ruled. He had a duty, then, to take care to avoid getting in accidents; he knew he was vulnerable, unlike the man having his first heart attack.

If you get kicked out of a bar, as opposed to your house, physically carried even, you're guilty of public drunkenness; did you really think you were going to sleep in the bar? Start the camera a little earlier; we go back in time to find the act which put you in the state of irresponsibility. You don't get off that easy; otherwise weakness would be an excuse.

Left on your own, you're overweight. Mindful eating and common sense have left you likelier to die young and hate yourself between now and then. Every day you will confront more situations like the ones you faced in the past, and your metabolism is slowing down to boot.

So what should you do? Keep driving like Mr. Decina and hope you'll beat the odds? Maybe he'll have a seizure while he's stopped at a light? Maybe you'll stop eating donuts without going on a diet?

But why in the world would you bet your life on it? That would be reckless indeed. It might even be enough to qualify as a depraved heart, which would bump you from involuntary manslaughter to second-degree murder.

I can't eat whatever I want. If I do, I will get fat. I wish that weren't true. Perhaps someday it won't be. But I doubt it. I think fudge tastes great. I love rich chocolate, bagels and cream cheese, any kind of bread, any kind of dessert . . . I like wine, peanuts, pizza . . . I don't want to think about this anymore. For me to eat without rules, particularly when my goal is to lose weight, is an act of reckless disregard for my own life not so different from Mr. Decina's decision to drive.

If someone told me tomorrow that I could eat anything I wanted and be slim and healthy, I would not eat oatmeal with skim milk for breakfast. Not even close. Waffles with syrup and butter one day, an apple pancake the next. I would not eat steamed vegetables for lunch or grilled chicken for dinner. Who's kidding whom?

This is why we have rules. This is why they ask you the question about your health on your license application, not after the accident. This is why we have diets, and why you have to go on one.

A diet is a set of rules, private law adopted by you and for you, in advance, when you're thinking straight and taking care. Whether it "works" or not depends on your commitment and on whether it's a smart diet. The commitment comes first. We're going to work out a contract, and you'll be asked to sign it—a set of promises you make and incentives we build in to make sure you keep to the rules you've adopted. Not that I don't trust you, but I'm a lawyer. Then, I'll present you with the plan. The secret, miracle plan, if you will . . .

I can't go into a donut shop and just order coffee. I can't buy one donut. It won't happen. The smell, the memory of my grandfather and going to Dunkin' Donuts as a kid, there it is. Now I could try to tell you or myself or whoever's listening later that it really isn't my fault, it's all about my childhood, but it won't matter to my hips because the damage will be done. And I could lie to myself and say I'll take the rest home, but I won't. There's only one answer.

I don't eat donuts. I don't buy donuts. I don't meet people for coffee at donut places. It's in my contract.

CHAPTER SIX

Making a Contract with Yourself

There is a fiction that "successful dieters"—those mythic people whose "case histories" I used to lie in bed at night and read—pick a diet, stay on it until all their excess weight is lost, and live happily ever after. In this fiction, they drop four or five pounds the first week, and one or two or three every week after that, until, say, in eight weeks, they've lost twenty pounds. You read about them and you say, I can do that. I said that a good deal. I never did it.

Studies suggest that people lose weight over time the same way we yo-yoers do—except they skip the up periods that cancel out all your efforts. You lose a few pounds, and then you plateau. That happens to everyone. It's what happens next that separates the successes from the failures. Failures begin heading back up again; successes keep going down. At the end of six months, the successes have had as many plateaus as the failures, but they kept heading down, instead of continually losing the same ten pounds over and over.

I figure over the course of my two decades of diet failure, I lost hundreds and hundreds of pounds. You probably have too. The problem was that in between losing those hundreds of pounds, in frustration, boredom, and so on, I gained even more.

So the answer is clear. Of course you can lose ten, twenty,

thirty, forty pounds. If you're a chronic dieter, you've already done that many times. You just have to avoid gaining it in between.

Three weeks is the minimum time that researchers say is necessary to begin establishing new patterns of behavior. You get used to things in three weeks.

Take a look at your calendar. How long can you commit to, right now? Don't say forever. Don't say six months.

For some people, one day is the only answer—one day at a time.

Look at the next three weeks. Is there anything in the next three weeks that you can't do and diet?

What is it? A pie-eating contest?

The most important thing you bring to any challenge is your commitment. Your determination to make something work is the single most important predictor of whether it will. You know that: we not only see it with our kids, we teach it to them, along with the importance of stretching themselves when they set their goals.

This is the moment of truth. You've spent enough money on diets that didn't work and diet books that you knew were stupid before you bought them.

Look in the mirror. There are worse things in the world than overeating. If you're happy with your weight, and your doctor is, God bless. If you're eating instead of doing something worse, to yourself or others, eat. If the next three weeks are full of impossible challenges that exhaust you simply to contemplate and you'd rather meet them than lose six to ten pounds, fine. It is a choice.

Make it now, when you're thinking straight, like Mr. Decina, when he gets in the car.

Either commit yourself to losing the weight, or stop carrying around all that baggage that says you should. Wanting to lose weight and not doing what it takes to succeed—particularly when you have the power to do so—is pointless, careless, and probably pretty stupid, wouldn't you say?

In the law, when two people make binding promises to each other, we call it a contract, and recommend that it be put in writing. It's true that a written contract helps settle conflicting claims if one or the other party breaches, but that's not what anyone wanted going in. We make contracts in the hope and expectation of fulfilling them. It is a statement of what we intend to do, a declaration of expectations and intentions.

When a legislature does this, or the public in a referendum, it's called a public law. When two parties do it in reaching an agreement, making a contract, settling a dispute out of court, it is private law. Instead of being bound by rules made by our representatives, we are bound by the rules we make ourselves. Formally, the promises in a contract are referred to as its terms. But they are really private rules—or for those who prefer, points of light, or my favorite, declarations of intent. You say you're going to change. Sure. Today's the first day of that new lifestyle. Right. I hope so, honestly I do. But you must see that yours is not a very persuasive case. I'm a lawyer. My client would fire me if I came back with nothing more than your promise that this time was going to be different.

I don't believe you. I think Susan's Miracle Diet is the smartest diet in the whole world, that it will train your brain, but I still don't believe you. I'm the lawyer for losing weight, after all, and "I'm starting a new diet (tomorrow)" is right up there with the check being in the mail and the rest. I want to see that promise actually fulfilled, which means I need much more than the vague boilerplate about how you're really going to try hard this time. Been there, done that.

We're not in court today. This is a negotiating session. We're negotiating your contract for the next three weeks, all the terms and conditions.

A contract is a mutual exchange of promises. On my side, on the side of losing weight, this is what I'm offering: If you follow my diet for the next three weeks, you will lose weight, feel better, look better, and like yourself more. If you can keep doing the same thing for somewhat longer, you will feel like a new person who has been given a new chance at life. You will be healthier, more attractive, more self-confident, and more likely to live a long, energetic, and productive life. You will also never be hungry.

For a low-fat diet and a program of moderate exercise, I'm offering a reduction in your risk of high blood pressure, heart disease, and colon cancer.

The question is, what are you offering? Declare your intentions. I want to see this contract fulfilled and, as my friend Bert, the fiercest contract negotiator in Hollywood, would explain to you, your goal in negotiating a contract is not to bind your side, but to keep the other side where you want them. In this case, on a diet.

The reason you're negotiating this contract and the reason you have to sign your name to it is to force you to go through the exercise that is essential to the success of any project, personal or professional. First, you come up with a plan. Second, you figure out how you're going to accomplish it. That's the part we dieters tend to skip, assuming that somehow, when we're facing the buffet table loaded with sweets, we will find sugar-free gelatin there, or the willpower to resist.

Wrong.

Before we start, pop quiz. On a scale of 1 to 10, how important is it for you to lose weight and get in shape? Don't think.

Give me a number. If it's lower than 9 (we'll reserve 10 for your family's good health, solvency, and world peace), you're not ready and you're going to fail. What's your favorite food? Isn't it at least an 8 on the pleasure scale? Thank you very much.

If I was called to go to Bosnia and settle the dispute, I would not turn the request down because I was on a diet. Assuming you're not called either, and that you can find a replacement for the pie-eating contest, is there anything/anyone else that you want to have stop you from losing weight and getting in shape for the next three weeks?

Open your calendar and look at the next three weeks. You've just been offered the deal of a lifetime and if you can find a way to fit it in, you will look back on this moment as one of those that changed your life. You know I'm right.

Can you say no? How can you possibly say no?

Look at your three weeks the way Bert would. You claim you're going on a diet for three weeks, but to be honest, there's not a whole lot in your past history to make us believe that it's very likely that you will. And the road ahead is full of land mines, the sort that have consistently undermined you in the past—family get-togethers, business trips, restaurant dinners, etc. There are basically two kinds of risks in life: the ones you can see coming, and the ones you can't. You can wait and see how you'll react when the risk arises and hope for the best, or you can decide now, pass a rule if you're a legislature, or put a provision in the contract if you're Bert. Don't drive when you're drunk and disabled. If travel is involved, here's how Mr. Cruise likes to go . . .

A good lawyer plans ahead for both kinds of risks, which is not easy. She has specific provisions to deal with the things she knows are coming, and general ones to be applied when the un-foreseeable happens. She wants everything she can in this con-tract to keep you to your promise. She'll build in steps, and conditions, and partial payments, the point of which is to antic-ipate in advance what could happen, and decide in advance what should if it does.

Besides, you have an advantage Bert doesn't have when he negotiates. You know the crazy person you're dealing with inside and out. You know where you need to tie her down, and get it in writing.

First, we need a message. The message is that one-sentence summary, that picture, that tune, that says it all, that tells you the answer even if we didn't see the question coming. Every success has a message; every failure is still trying to figure it out. This diet, this last diet, needs a message.

It's what you refer to when you're between two rules, two diets, a rock and a hard place. It's the first thing you think of if you think of breaking a rule, ignoring a pledge, undercutting your commitment. It's the sentence at the top of your contract.

The way you figure out the message, in addition to the can-didate consulting his or her views, beliefs, and principles, of course, is by testing it on people. You see how they react to the words, the idea, the ad, the speech, the event; you see what works and what doesn't. You measure response. These days, you can give people buttons to point, pressure points, all kinds of things that measure reaction.

Think about your mission. Think about what makes this time different. Pick a cliché. The reason they're clichés is because they work. Here are some that have stuck in my head: "It's just food." "No more excuses." "No one's going to like you if you don't like yourself." "Enough with your mother already." "If in doubt, no." "Only you can save yourself."

Imagine a time, sometime in the future, when something totally unexpected happens, and your first thought is that you want a double sausage sandwich, what do you want your second thought to be?

[WRITE IT IN BIG LETTERS HERE.]

When you get tired of it, change it.

1. I promise to follow Susan's Miracle Diet for twenty-one days as prescribed. I promise to devote one hour every day, for each of the next twenty-one days, to exercise and self-renewal. I will mark the hours on the calendar right now.

Write it down now. On your regular calendar, which you have to look at every single day. You give me twenty-one days, and then you can decide for the rest of your life. No restaurant lunches or dinners in the first three days. You'll understand later, believe me. I'll insist on it.

Also, Bert is insisting on that hour a day. Every day. He knows you said this was important, a 9 and all that, but as I say, he's a lawyer. An hour a day is a measure of importance. That ensures you have time to exercise, and a little time for rewards. It makes dieting more attractive. One less hour of everything else. You have to mark it now.

If you work, mark it on your calendar as CD—Client Development. You're working developing your most important client, yourself. I learned this trick from a girlfriend, who wanted to get to Mommy and Me classes with her youngest, and knew if she marked them as that on her calendar, they would disappear. So she marked them as client development, and when people would call or check her book, there it would be. Mommy and Me, they would've booked a meeting. Client Development is something everyone considers important.

If you work at home, mark it RN. If anyone asks, tell them it's short for one of your newest volunteer projects, in the health field, perhaps they'd like to volunteer with you? Sadly, that will probably end the conversation.

What does CD—RN really stand for?

Corpus Delecti—Right Now.

2. I promise to plan in advance for every event that involves eating over the next twenty-one days, and to consider my diet as a valid and legitimate basis to decide not to go somewhere.

Look at all the events scheduled for the next three weeks at which food or drink will be served. If there are events that you can't get through without blowing your diet, give them fair warning and tell them now that you aren't coming. You do not have to expose yourself to superhuman temptation if you can avoid it. Your diet is more important than whether someone's feelings will be hurt if you skip a family gathering in which overeating has been a steady pattern for thirty years. Later on, when you're thin, see if you can get through it on diet tonic water. Now, don't go. Promise me you won't.

My friend Mary is a nutritionist. She is healthy and smart. She's the type who can eat half a sandwich. But her husband told me a little secret. He's not allowed to bring chocolate into the house. Mary can't resist it. So she doesn't have it around. It's Mr. Decina all over again. Avoid temptations you find it difficult to resist. If you don't want to drive home from the bar drunk, you shouldn't drive there. If you can't go to a bar without drinking and you're trying not to drink, don't go to a bar. When you drive there, you've made the decision to drive drunk later. Decisions have consequences. You are responsible for considering them. Of course you might have sipped soda water all night in the bar, but how often does that happen? Certainly a lot less often than Mr. Decina's seizures. A diet imposes on you a duty of care to avoid situations where you'll be unconscious later.

If you can't get through the bridal shower without eating— don't go. Tell them it's a health problem—yours. If there are people you're supposed to have dinner with where the only pleasure is eating, don't go. If there's a restaurant with a dessert you can't resist, pick another restaurant. If going to your mother's makes you eat, meet her at the mall. If you are promising to do something you've never done before, tell me exactly how it is you think you'll pull it off this time.

And remember, you are entitled to make your preference the group preference for the next three weeks. It might get to be a habit.

For goodness' sake, can't I at least have a good time at a cocktail party?

Sure. What would a good time be?

A few drinks, a few of those little pass-around hors d'oeuvres . . .

A few? Do you mean one or two or four or six or eight or ten of those little pastry treats? Have you ever had one or two, or does one or two become three or four and then another drink and a few peanuts while you wait for the drink and some chips and now you're so thirsty and some- one passes you a pizza and cheese and chips and onion dip . . . And now how do you feel? Are you the life of the party? Are you brimming with self-confidence, full of energy, ready to woo, win, charm, or do whatever you choose? No, you're thinking about getting your coat so you can go home and take off the skirt that is suddenly incredibly tight around the waist, and you're feeling hot and full of potato chips, not confidence . . .

But it's only once in a while. Why not say, "The heck with the guilt, I'm going to enjoy myself for one night." So I'll wear elastic pants.

Sure. And what are you going to wear the day after?

Most of us diet failures don't blow it because of the big events. I forgot to eat at my own wedding, and ended up eating a peanut butter and jelly sandwich left behind by a four-year-old guest after the caterers had packed up. If you want a piece of cake at the wedding, and it's not going to lead you to eat everything in sight, fine. But one piece. Decide that in advance. That's on your diet, not off it. It's not a green light for lunacy at the sweet table.

Here's the problem. Events aren't the only obstacle to a successful diet; in my case, and I go to a lot of events, they've never been big problems. Usually, there's something else to do at an event, even if eating is its focus, which it often isn't. In fact, if eating isn't the focus, you don't have to eat at all (which I find possible, as opposed to eating just a piece of a muffin . . .); even if eating is the focus, like lunch, you can talk, or listen, or do whatever it is you came to do other than eat (assuming you're not a restaurant critic). Events are easy compared to people and things. If I gave myself permission in advance to eat at events, and then added in the havoc that people and life can bring, I wouldn't be on a diet. I'd be on a plan to gain weight. That's how I gained 110 pounds in two pregnancies.

3. I promise not to let other people divert me from my goal. I promise to adopt and abide by rules of engagement, attached to this agreement as an addendum, in dealing with the people I will see in the next three weeks. I will lie to them (so long as it doesn't endanger my health, of course) rather than invite even well-meaning sabotage.

People, particularly people you love, are probably the biggest obstacle to a successful diet. Some of them want you to succeed and some of them want you to fail. It hardly matters; you'll eat more if you listen to any of them.

It is tempting to try to lose weight for someone—to do it, say, for a special man in your life. Tempting, but ultimately stupid. Maintaining a good relationship with a man is hard enough without inserting your diet into the equation. If you diet for someone, it only follows that you'll eat for them too—at least when you get mad at them, which you are almost certain to do, since they are after all depriving you of one of life's great pleasures.

It's hard enough to lose weight in order to lose weight without loading a relationship on top of it.

You can lose weight because of your love for someone—I love my kids, and I use them freely in the case—but they're not the ones who decided I should diet. I love the fact that people sometimes figure I'm the trophy wife, and that my husband can't believe the figure on his bride, but I didn't go on a diet for him. I went on it for me. You have to.

As for the people who want you to fail, there are probably more of them than you'd care to believe. Everyone will tell you that what you're doing is unhealthy, wrong, ill-fated, foolish, that you look drawn, too thin, not enough iron, not enough fat, whatever it is you're doing will not be as good as what they've heard about or are about to try. They will undermine your confidence in your plan, your approach, and yourself. They love you. But the prospect that you really can lose weight and get in shape is incredibly threatening to everyone who can't. They do not want to hear about how well you are doing. They need you to fail, not because they hate you, but because that way, they won't have to give up donuts. Some of the thin ones don't want you to get thin, because then it will matter more to them that you're smarter, or prettier, or have blonder hair. They like being the thin one. For some, it's all they have.

Perhaps there is someone in your circle who is the perfect diet companion. Probably not. There are no doubt a good many people to whom you should simply say nothing at all. While I was dieting, I had a simple rule: I discussed it with people on a "need to know" basis. The waiter needs to know that you want the sauce on the side. If your mother asks why, just say, "That way I can dip. Gee, your hair looks nice, Mom. Is someone new doing it?"

Most people are either thin and not interested in diets, or about to eat a sausage sandwich and not eager to hear why they shouldn't. The belief that it is "impossible to lose weight" becomes a mantra for women who are used to accomplishing the impossible, and being cheerily told that they're wrong is something better accomplished by a stranger on the printed page than one-on-one with your loved ones. In other words, just because you love them, don't try to convince them to go on a diet with you. Don't try to change their minds. It's enough work to change your own.

If you want to discuss your diet, if you want to talk and get support, join Weight Watchers, Overeaters Anonymous, or other groups of like-minded strangers trying to help each other. As for your friends and family, you need to plan as carefully how you want to deal with them as you do the events on your schedule.

You need to adopt rules of engagement that tell you how you're going to deal with and respond to people. You can use humor (when people trying to urge steak on me say, "But don't you eat meat?" I sometimes smile and say, "Only from . . ." Fill it in. Make it funny); you can use avoidance (a new project at work has left you unbelievably busy for the next three weeks); you can lie and say you've already eaten; you can deceive and wear extra bright lipstick with the relatives most likely to say you're looking drawn.

What you should never do is ask someone else's permission to do what you have the right and power to do, or make your ability to do it conditioned on something they think, do, or say. No one should have so much power and if they do (so it goes), the least you can do is not make it easier for them to undermine you.

Make a list of the people you will be seeing over the next three weeks. Consider what context you're seeing them in, whether they normally drive you to donuts, or stress you to sausage sandwiches. See more people for breakfast (easy, fruit and coffee or hot cereal and tea or whatever) and fewer for dinner, which is longer, making it harder (particularly with drinks) not to overeat. Meet people for a walk. Tell them you're busy for lunch. Do work instead (the phone doesn't ring as much). See people in places where you diet best, which may not be your mother's kitchen.

4. Within the limits of health, morals, and fiscal responsibility, I promise to do whatever else I want for the next twenty-one days.

Things happen, and they will continue to happen for the next three weeks. You won't get the job, he won't call for a date, you won't get in where you want, something will get dumped on you, there will be bills you don't expect, bad news about an old friend, sickness in the family, the stuff of life . . .

What makes eating so useful is it fills so many needs at once:

a treat, a comfort, an activity, a distraction, a reward, a punishment; there's almost nothing you can't get, emotionally, from the grocery store or the refrigerator/freezer.

You need to give yourself permission to do other things when you need them. You need other sources of comfort, support, pleasure, satisfaction, and relaxation, if you're about to lose food. It isn't that food is so great—it really isn't a reward, in the long run. But in the short run, it fills the space.

Why did he write that? I once asked my husband about a particularly mean and gratuitous column. Space to fill, he answered, and once I was a columnist, I understood. Why did you eat that? I would sometimes ask myself. Filled the space. It was there.

Make a list of the rewards you plan to give yourself as you progress through the next twenty-one days. They can be things, time, space: a book, a massage, a half-day for yourself, a new bra and underwear; for me, an hour in the aisles of Marshalls or Ross Dress for Less is pure relaxation. What days are you going? Plenty of rewards for you. The next time anything bad happens, immediately buy yourself a new lipstick. The next time you get incredibly angry and are ready to eat everything in sight, go get your nails done (always a surefire food-stopper).

5. I promise to change my clothes when I come home from work or errands at the end of the day, put on something comfortable, and spend one minute taking a deep breath and remembering the message of my diet before I enter the kitchen for the first time.

Under the first amendment, the government isn't supposed to tell you what to say. But it can impose time, place, and manner restrictions on your speech. Those restrictions tend to be controversial, often ending up in the Supreme Court, because everyone understands that regulating the time, place, and manner of speaking has a direct and incontrovertible effect on the speech itself.

Eating is the same way. Diets will tell you what to eat. That's never the problem. It's when, where, and how that does most of us in. So we use that to our advantage. It's not enough to agree to what you are going to eat. You also have to change how you eat. Don't worry: this is really just about sitting down and getting comfortable.

Most of us are boringly similar: we break our diets at night, alone, standing up or driving, eating from containers, other people's plates, or directly from the refrigerator. On average, people consume 70 percent of their calories after five P.M. Virtually every woman I know tells me she gets in trouble the minute she gets home. Relax when you get home. Change your clothes. Put some moisturizer on your hands and face (who wants to start messing with food when you're creaming your hands?). Go for a walk if it's still light out. Then start the dinner.

6. I promise not to go to the grocery store on my way home from work or at the end of the day. I will get up early and go before work instead. If I stop for take-out food on the way home, I will not buy enough for the neighbors.

I love the grocery store. I used to go there at night, on my way home from work, and see all these other working women there buying junk they would never buy at seven-thirty in the morning. We end up eating our way up and down the aisles, only to realize it's always later than we think, so we pick up some of that nice, practically poisonous orange chicken (a day's calories in a small carton) to bring home to the kids.

If you want to stop for thirty minutes of relaxation on your way home from work, go shoe shopping, go try on fancy underwear, go buy some flowers, or just amble up and down the aisles of your local discount bed-and-bath store, which has all the same satisfactions as grocery shopping (you're getting things you need for the family, not—heaven forbid—little luxuries for yourself) without the calories. Do not go to the grocery store. It's just asking for trouble.

If you need things for supper, buy what you need for supper. If you're picking up take-out, only get enough for the people who are eating. If you are the only one eating, buy one portion, not two. You are not shopping for the neighbors. They will not stop by unannounced and also want pasta and basil. You do not need cheese and crackers to serve to them. You cannot eat what you do not buy. From that it follows that you should not buy what you don't want to eat, and you should not shop when you are most likely to do so. At night. After five P.M. The high-crime time.

7. I promise to stop eating every night by 8:30 at the latest on weekdays and 9:30 on weekends.

Curfews work. Keep kids off the street at night, and they can't get into trouble. Keep you from eating at night, and you'll lose weight. Prime time starts, you stop eating. This is the easiest way to lose weight—because eating at night is the easiest way to gain it.

Use a ritual to stop eating for the night. Drink a cup of herbal tea, or good coffee or decaf.

Say a prayer. Answer the nightly interrogatories. Put a fresh coat of topcoat on your nails, which will be ruined completely if you mess them up eating. Turn off the light in the kitchen. Declare it closed. Tell anyone else in the family that they can serve themselves, and also bring you tea, and also clean up after themselves. It is good for them, and you deserve it.

8. I promise to write a memorandum to the file every night for the next twenty-one days. I will not lie. I will not be too busy. I will exercise one additional hour for every day I miss.

I always used to lie in those food journals they gave me at the Diet Center. But there's no point in lying to yourself, particularly when it carries a penalty of an extra hour of exercise. The reason I would lie is because I didn't want to face myself. The reason you have to keep a journal is because the only way you're going to remake yourself is by facing yourself.

I'm less interested in learning what you ate than the Diet Center ladies were, particularly on days when I told you and that's what you ate. Every single diet book that is even semi-intelligent encourages you to write down what you eat. If we could only pay attention, this would be so easy. If wishes were horses, beggars would ride. I still don't do it, even if I should.

But I do make notes about what I'm thinking, what I'm feeling and learning, and that is even more important. If you're not thinking your way through the next twenty-one days, you won't learn anything, or change. But how do you make people think? In classes, we do it by calling on people, never announcing in advance who it will be, so that everyone must be prepared. If you don't brief the case the night before, it's at your own risk, because the person called on could be you.

You don't need me to call on you. Call on yourself. Every morning you check your calendar. What's today's plan? How are you going to do it? Pick a mantra for the day—a cliché to carry with you. Confirm your exercise schedule. Check the paper for underwear sales.

Every night, open up your journal and write a memo to the file. Dictate it. Do it on your computer. Do it in a pretty blank book that you bought on the way home from work instead of the sausage sandwich. I've already given you some special questions for the different stages of your diet, but these are ones to think of at any time:

> ➤ Did you take good care of your body today? How?
> ➤ Did you eat what you planned and intended to eat?
> ➤ Did you exercise as you planned and intended to?
> ➤ How did you feel afterward?
> ➤ Was there any part of it you enjoyed? Which?
> ➤ How many times did you face down temptation today? How did you do it?
> ➤ How many times did you consciously make the case for losing weight to yourself?
> ➤ Which arguments worked?
> ➤ Did you cheat?
> ➤ What did you have?
> ➤ Did you stop or keep going?
> ➤ When you did stop, how?
> ➤ Did you do anything truly stupid and/or dangerous to yourself which should send you to a doctor? GO.
> ➤ Assuming you didn't, what's your best analysis of why you cheated?
> ➤ How do you plan to cope better in the future?
> ➤ Did cheating help?
> ➤ Did it make you feel worse?
> ➤ Are you bored? Is there something you crave? What? What do you plan to do about it? How do you intend to address the craving?
> ➤ Of the things you ate today, what did you enjoy most?

What did you enjoy not at all? Did you waste calories? On what?

➤ What nice thing did you do for yourself today other than eat?

➤ What is your plan for tomorrow?

Say a blessing. You are one of the luckiest people in the world. And go to sleep.

9. I promise to make the case for myself before I violate this contract, to premeditate and deliberate before I violate the rules of Susan's Miracle Diet. I will not eat standing up, straight from the container, or in the car.

A promise not to cheat isn't worth much to me, but a promise to do so only deliberately has a chance of deterring you. If you have to think before you cheat, if you have to make the case for yourself and then do yourself in, you're less likely to do it. If you have to sit down and cheat, and you do it deliberately and premeditatedly, it's not cheating. It's enjoying a special treat, which you don't do very often, and certainly should enjoy when you do.

9a. If I cheat, I will not use it as an excuse to derail my diet. I will accept the consequences and resume my strict adherence to the twenty-one-day plan.

Speaks for itself. The words "since I've already blown it, I might as well . . ." should never come out of your mouth.

10. I promise to try to remember that this is a good thing I'm doing, a positive intention, not a terrible deprivation. When I'm feeling

sorry for myself, I will smile for one minute and make the case for myself.

Your body chemistry changes when you smile. Makes sense, doesn't it? Smile right now. Feel your body change. Why not use this to your advantage? Remember your message. Use it as a mantra. You are doing this because you want to. The hardest part is the moment you are resisting a treat. It passes really quickly—as would the treat, right on to your hips, if you ate it. Close your eyes for thirty seconds and it's gone. That can be as true for the craving as it is for the treat.

11. I promise to devote all of my energies, attention, and determination to making my diet work. I alone take responsibility for making it work.

Signed and sworn on this _____ day of _____, 199_

HAVE YOU ALREADY FOUND YOUR OWN MIRACLE DIET?

If you've found a diet that works for you, and it's healthy, you can SKIP the next two chapters.

Any diet will work if it results in reduced calorie intake. If you get basic nutritional needs satisfied in the process, it's a healthy diet to boot. The critical question, beyond that, is how hard it is for you to follow.

Different diets "work" for different people. My friend Leslie swears that Barry Sears' Zone diet is the best diet she's ever been on. The diet, which emphasizes combining protein and carbohydrate blocks, has been much criticized in the scientific community, but it's clear, at least in Leslie's case, why all of that is irrelevant. Whether or not eating protein and carbohydrate in blocks has a special effect, it clearly leads you to eat more protein and less pasta. You'll lose weight. Leslie, who was eating very little protein, is eating twice as much, feels stronger, and swears by the Zone. At least until she gets sick of it.

My friend Patty thought the Zone was the worst. She loves carrots. Carrots aren't allowed. "What kind of diet doesn't let me eat carrots?" she asks, and it's perfectly clear that whatever kind it is, it's not the right one for her. (Susan's Miracle Diet lets you eat carrots, by the way.)

One of the things you'll learn from my Miracle Diet is how to figure out what the best diet is for you. The best diet for you is the one that, by the end, gives you a better understanding of what the choices and tradeoffs are and a more objective insight into your own responses to different regimes. There's no point wasting discipline when you don't need to, forcing yourself to give up carrots if you love them.

Unfortunately, even if you find the perfect diet, there will still come a time when a cupcake is courting you, a sundae makes eyes at you across the counter, and you will need to make the case for yourself. Even the perfect diet doesn't guarantee perfect compliance all the time.

In short, if you've got the perfect diet, let me help you stick to it. And if you get bored with your perfect diet, you can always try my Miracle.

Lawyer Alert

I am not a doctor. I am not a nutritionist.

Do not do some stupid thing and then come along and say "I" told you to do it. As a matter of law, I'm telling you right here: Don't listen to me. You decide. You're responsible. That's what I'm telling you.

Make your doctor your partner in this effort.

If you have an eating disorder, you should get help from a doctor. I can't even tell you where the line is between cheating and bingeing, between dieters and people with eating disorders.

(Women think three donuts is a binge, men six. Can you imagine eating five donuts and calling it a snack?)

If you're in doubt, what do you think? Get help. If it were your kid, pet, aunt, mother, would you get help?

It's not your fault that you're sick. It's not a sign that you are a weak, foolish person. When you're sick, you need medicine and help to get better.

In this case, there is no argument for the other side.

CHAPTER SEVEN

Susan's Miracle Diet

Diets are not magic. They work not because there's some secret science to eating beef stew on Tuesdays, as Jenny Craig used to require, or cabbage soup, the foundation of the Not-the-Heart Association diet, but because any set of rules that gets you to eat no more than 1,000 to 1,500 calories a day (and move more) will cause you to lose weight. No magic.

We all know that.

The greatest accomplishment of a diet is generally what it keeps you away from. Only eat hot cereal for breakfast. OK. Truth is, depending upon what kind you choose, cold cereal can be just as nutritious. But it's not the cold cereal that the hot cereal requirement is really keeping you away from: it's the Belgian waffle with whipped cream, the blueberry muffin, etc.

We know that too.

You don't need to restrict yourself to hot cereal if you feel like cold cereal to lose weight. Most nutritionists would tell you not to; avoid rigid rules, eat like a diabetic does, allowing yourself a specified number of portions of the different food groups, restricting fats, and paying special care to portion size with complex carbohydrates. You can't argue with that advice. The only problem is that it doesn't seem to work, and no one is even interested in hearing it.

Don't get me wrong. Information is important. If you don't know this you should. Foods belong to groups. Fat is not only bad for your arteries, it contains the most concentrated calories, which is why a little bit adds a lot to your hips. Conventional wisdom says you should restrict fat to somewhere between 10 and 30 percent of your caloric intake, and if you aim for 0 percent, you'll end up at 10 percent. Knowing all this should help you lose weight. But it doesn't. Such a pity.

There are dozens of very good books full of sensible advice about eating more fruits and vegetables, cooking the healthy way, and restricting fats. But most of them can't begin to compete, sales-wise, with the gimmicky diets that tell you to drink nothing but juice for three days, or to pick your diet according to your blood type / horoscope / mother's maiden name.

Are we crazy?

No.

We can't be.

We laugh at ourselves when we go on these crazy diets, and are careful about whom we tell. We know it's silly, but we do it anyway.

So what can we learn from our attraction to these gimmicks and fads that force you to give up things you don't need to give up and treat food like it's magic or evil when it's just food? And, even more important, how can you make that attraction work for you?

Here is what I have learned:

> At the beginning of a diet, I can do anything.
> Sometimes drastic changes are easier to make than small ones.
> Novelty is an enormous attraction of its own. For the first few days anyway, a new diet is almost always eas-

ier than an old one, even if it's more restrictive, defies common sense, and is scientifically laughable.

➤ We are not worried about losing weight too fast. I think the good guys and girls should stop using that admonition in their warning against fad diets; it only makes them look more attractive.

➤ Finally, however much I may tell you that dieting is up to you and you have to take responsibility, we want someone else to tell us what to do. We don't want to be told to just do it. We want to be told what to do.

Now, I could make the case that all those responses which virtually everyone reading this will recognize are misguided and inappropriate; that we shouldn't be attracted to novelty; shouldn't be willing to take orders from others; that we shouldn't feel so gratified by that first initial weight loss.

But why? You don't want to hear that. You already know it and it doesn't help.

If you're going to change the way you diet, it won't be just because I tell you to. Lots of people have told you to. You've told yourself to. Doesn't work.

Jujitsu is in order. Instead of attacking your desire for novelty, I'm going to play to it. Instead of deriding you because I know you'll be bored in a matter of days, I'm going to take advantage of that. I'm going to tell you what to do. I don't just have one diet. I have four. I made them all up. Nutritionally, they're a little better than most of their competitors. But that wasn't the driving force.

The challenge I set for myself was to use a few basic diets to structure your thinking about diets, to take you from crash dieting to dieting like a grown-up, from looking for answers elsewhere to finding them from within. We train your brain to take over from mine. Sometimes the only way to make the case is to live it.

As I said earlier, I decided to call my diet Susan's Miracle Diet, so that it would feel comfortable in the bookstore alongside the other miracle, secret, and wonder diets. It is the product of twenty-five years of self-experimentation, and endless hours examining all the books that I wasted money on over the years. In my lawyerlike way, I've approached diets the way I would statutory schemes, breaking them into categories, figuring out which ones taught me things and which ones were a waste of time, and what it was they taught me, and why it was they failed. I've created my own set of doctrines in an effort to understand what makes diets attractive, what it is we are looking for in them, and what it is we need.

It's sort of like common law, only the subject is dieting. Reading each case and fitting them together, judges and scholars strive to learn the lessons of the past, to follow what was right and true and discard what was wrong and misguided, to keep moving forward, applying principle to situations, using the best at hand. I decided to make my case in a series of diets. Or as diet doctors and law professors of old always used to say, just do it and you'll understand later.

Days 1–3: Miracle Diet Number One a.k.a. "The Bad Girl's Diet"

Health Alert: You will lose weight fast. Too fast. (Scared, aren't you?)

This is a crash diet. I have tried every crash diet in the world. This is the easiest one I have tried, and also the only one that ever taught me anything useful. It is not the Heart Association diet. It is not even the Not-the-Heart Association diet; the Xeroxed version I got was full of fat and salt and cholesterol, which is not the way to diet, even when you're crash dieting. This one's better. Nonetheless, it would not be good for you to live on this diet forever, because it doesn't have enough protein and calcium, but not to worry; I've never met anybody who could.

Make a pot of cabbage soup in the morning, or the night before. It must be ready when you need it. You can bring it to work and heat it up. Or you can keep the pot on the stove all day, the way I do, which is sort of soothing.

> **Breakfast:** An orange, a grapefruit, an apple, or half a cantaloupe—or all of them if you're that hungry
>
> **Between breakfast and lunch:** Two cups herbal tea, a peach, a nectarine, or a tangerine—or all of them
>
> **Lunch:** As much cabbage soup as you want. If you add Equal, it will actually satisfy your sweet tooth—if it's hurting. (Or as my friend Skip says, "With Equal, I could live on this.")
>
> **Between lunch and dinner:** Two cups herbal tea
>
> **Dinner:** As much cabbage soup as you want
>
> **After dinner:** Two cups herbal tea
>
> **Throughout the day:** Coffee, tea, diet soda—as much as you want

If you get hungry, you can eat more cabbage soup, or celery or carrot sticks.

If you're still hungry, add nonfat plain yogurt to the cabbage soup and check out a good book while riding the exercise bike.

Unlimited sugar-free diet gelatin is okay too.

We cleanse, rotate, and jump right in.

SUSAN'S BASIC CABBAGE SOUP

1 head cabbage (green, red, or mixed), chopped
2 cans fat-free, low-salt or salt-free chicken or vegetable
    broth, or homemade stock, skimmed of fat
1 28-ounce can low-salt chopped tomatoes
1 28-ounce can low-salt stewed tomatoes
4 or 5 celery stalks, cut up
2 onions, cut up
2 or 3 carrots
    Spices

Put in a large soup pot the cabbage, broth, tomatoes, celery, onion, and carrots. Toss in whatever spices you can find around, add water to cover, bring all to a boil, then cover and simmer for a couple of hours. For a richer soup, add a little can of salt-free tomato puree or some fat-free tomato sauce. Sweeten with Equal.

For connoisseurs, Marty's seasoning suggestions and Grandma Dorothy's better, more complicated recipe for cabbage soup are at the back of the book.

SPECIAL RULES FOR MIRACLE DIET NUMBER ONE

These are the first three days of your last diet. It is important to succeed. This is the easiest crash diet in the world, *unless* you try to do it under impossible conditions. Then you will fail and blame me. No way. No restaurants on cabbage soup days, except for breakfast, if necessary, for fruit and coffee. If it's a work day, bring a big, huge container of your cabbage soup, eat it at your desk, and tell everyone you're too busy to waste time at a restaurant. Better yet, if you can, declare it a personal day, clean your closets, get a massage, and have soup. (I say things like this, but in all honesty, I never do them; I do, however, have a big thermos.)

I'm convinced one of the reasons so many busy people swear by juice fasts is because it gives them a reason to slow down for the day, to meditate, to be mindful, to reconnect—because you can't run around at a hundred miles an hour if you're only drinking juice. I can't get through a day on just juice—it's much harder than cabbage soup and fruit—and I can't slow down . . . But if you can, why not do it with fruit and less salty, better-tasting cabbage soup? Just don't get too comfortable.

MEMORANDUM TO THE FILE

At the end of every day, write a memo to the file answering the key questions of the day.

Susan, come on. . . .

What? I know you're busy, you don't want to make this your life's work, you just want to lose weight . . . but remember, this is a 9 on the 1 to 10 scale; we've already had this conversation.

The lawyer for losing weight is sending you nightly interrogatories that need to be answered. Forces you to pay attention. Writing down what you're thinking makes you think harder.

I'll ask some of the night's questions, but remember, we're all on the same team in this one. We have one goal. I'm not looking to trip you up, and you're not looking to prove that my diet doesn't work. We both want you to lose weight. Defeat will be the orphan. As for success, there'll be plenty of credit to go around.

Which is to say, before you answer the questions, write some. There is a great story about the final exam in a property class at Harvard Law School. The famous but supposedly lazy professor waited until the very last minute to write his exam, which can be a time-consuming and tedious affair, requiring the invention of some long and convoluted hypothetical in which every issue of the course is so cleverly hidden that even very smart students who have studied unbelievably hard will miss half of them. Finally, the professor turned in two sentences:

1. Assuming the course to be the same, please write the question for next year's exam.
2. Answer it.

End of exam.

In each set of questions I'll give you from now on, the last one will always be the same. What question should I have asked? Answer it.

➤ Why are you doing this?
➤ How do you feel?
➤ How do you want to feel?
➤ Is it worth it?
➤ List all the reasons why.
➤ Were you full?
➤ Did you stuff yourself?
➤ How much of your day did you spend thinking about food?
➤ What did you think about?
➤ Did you feel deprived?
➤ Did you fight back against feeling deprived?
➤ How many times did you consciously and deliberately make the case to yourself for losing weight?
➤ Did you do it at least once every hour?
➤ If not, was it because you weren't tempted to cheat, or because you gave in?
➤ In what ways do you feel better today than yesterday?
➤ Was it easier than you expected?
➤ How many minutes were actually difficult?

➤ How'd you get through them?

➤ How many times today did you remind yourself you were on a diet?

➤ How many times did you remind yourself why you were on a diet?

➤ What nice thing did you do for yourself today?

➤ What's your reward for doing so well?

➤ Did you buy caraway seeds to put in the cabbage soup for tomorrow? Why not?

➤ What question should I have asked?

You may feel today like you could live on this forever (I hope) or at least for the duration of this diet. But you can't. You won't. That's why there are new diet books every year. Maybe this week, maybe next, you will start eating other things—and it may include everything in sight. Instead of a success, this diet, like every other one, will have been a failure.

Take the three-day victory and keep going. Don't push it. The goal is to keep winning. Miracle Diet Number One is very easy when you're on your own, not meeting people for dinner, not in business lunches where it's hard to take out your Tupperware (order the fruit salad instead, and eat your cabbage soup for breakfast). You will wake up one morning and not want to face the sight of cabbage soup, only to find yourself stuck in traffic in front of a donut shop. No way. You need another miracle.

Days 4–8: Miracle Diet Number Two a.k.a. "The Hollywood Diet"

Diets like this are often named after the place where the author lives. I live in Hollywood, the most diverse and interesting part of Los Angeles, which means this must be the Hollywood Miracle.

I tell you exactly what to do. I've got a very simple, basic, five-day all-you-can-eat menu plan, the product of my years of experience and months of work cataloguing, typologizing, trying, and inventing diets. The five easiest diet days I can think of. You get to see how painless five days of dieting can be, how much you can eat, how well you can do. And before you have a chance to get bored, or show me how you could do it better, you get a chance to do just that.

Breakfast (every day)
A grapefruit, an orange, or half a cantaloupe; one slice
   whole wheat/gluten bread or 75-calorie Back East bialy
Coffee or tea

Lunch I
Broiled chicken breast sliced in a large tossed salad with
   tomatoes and diet dressing
Coffee, tea, or diet soda

Dinner I
Fish or shellfish
Steamed vegetables, as much as you want
Sliced strawberries or other fruit
Coffee, tea, or diet soda

Lunch II
Fruit salad
Coffee, tea, or diet soda

Dinner II   Roast turkey breast or grilled turkey breast
   burgers
Large salad, as much as you want

Diet gelatin with fruit
Coffee, tea, or diet soda

Lunch III
White tuna (packed in water)
Vegetable salad
Grapefruit or melon
Coffee, tea, or diet soda

Dinner III
Turkey breast meatloaf
Steamed spinach
Salsa
Coffee, tea, or diet soda

Lunch IV
Egg Beaters or egg white omelette, made with peppers,
  onions, tomatoes, and/or other vegetables, and nonfat
  ricotta cheese
Baked apple
Coffee, tea, or diet soda

Dinner IV
Roast, barbecued, or baked chicken (white meat only,
  no skin)
Steamed vegetables, as much as you want
Salad with Marty's Miracle Dressing (see page 187)
Coffee, tea, or diet soda

Lunch V
Fruit plate
Coffee, tea, or diet soda

Dinner V
Isabel's Sloppy Burgers (see page 189) or spaghetti squash
  with fat-free turkey and tomato sauce

Salad, as much as you want
Baked apple
Coffee, tea, or diet soda

Looks pretty good, doesn't it? You will not be hungry. For five days, pretend it's magic. Don't change anything. Just do it.

SPECIAL RULES FOR MIRACLE DIET NUMBER TWO

Eat until you're full, but don't stuff yourself.

Between meals, you can have all the celery, cucumber, or carrot sticks you want.

Only low-calorie, fat-free dressings may be used.

No alcohol, lots of water. This is not a philosophical issue for me, but a calorie one. There are two problems with alcoholic beverages. One, they have calories. Two, they weaken your resistance and lead you to consume even more calories. Stop drinking for two weeks. It's an amazingly major step toward losing weight. In the third week, you can start drinking again—but you'll have to give up something for every drink you consume. If you can't stop drinking for two weeks, it's probably worth focusing some attention on what that means, maybe even before you start dieting.

The only vegetables you can't eat are corn, potatoes, avocados, peas, and acorn or winter squash (other than spaghetti squash).

Everything should be grilled, baked, broiled, or otherwise cooked without butter, oil, or anything else that would add fat or calories. Spray the pan with Pam or oil spray but keep away from the real thing. Vegetables just soak it up.

Use white chicken and turkey; buy the extra lean, not the lean; it's worth the money when you get more food for your caloric investment. You can substitute tofu and legumes for all my protein. But if you're not a vegetarian, go for the chicken and fish.

MEMORANDUM TO THE FILE

How'm I doing? as New York City mayor Ed Koch used to say. I must have read and tried a million different menus to come up with these, but I bet you can come up with better ones.

> ➤ Tell me what you like best about each day, and what is hardest.
> ➤ Which combinations work for you?
> ➤ Which is your favorite day?
> ➤ What is the easiest part of this diet for you?
> ➤ How do you feel when you go to bed at night?
> ➤ How do you feel when you wake up in the morning?
> ➤ Are you used to eating this much protein?
> ➤ Do you feel stronger?
> ➤ What do you miss most? (If the answer is chocolate, add diet hot chocolate to your menu.)
> ➤ Are you ready to start making some decisions for yourself?
> ➤ Are you ready for some electives?

Days 9–13: Miracle Diet Number Three a.k.a. "The Fresser"

Fresser is Yiddish for "big eater." The fresser sandwich is always the biggest on the menu. You can eat the turkey fresser, just hold the bread and the mayonnaise.

Eat all you want, whenever you want, but only of the following:

Vegetables

Artichokes
Asparagus
Broccoli
Cabbage
Carrots
Cauliflower
Celery
Cucumbers
Eggplant
Fennel
Green beans
Kale
Lettuce
Mushrooms
Okra
Onions
Peppers
Spaghetti squash
Spinach
Sprouts
Summer squash
Tomatoes

Fruit

Apples
Berries
Cantaloupe
Grapefruit
Mango
Nectarines
Oranges
Papaya
Peaches
Pears
Pineapple
Plums

Protein

Chicken, white meat
Egg whites or Egg Beaters
Fish or shellfish,
   low-fat only
Tofu
Turkey, white meat

Miscellaneous

Broth, chicken or
   vegetable, fat-free
Cheese, cottage, or ricotta,
   nonfat
Milk, nonfat
Mustard
Salad dressing, fat-free
Salsa
Tomato sauce,
   fat- and sugar-free

Beverages

Coffee
Diet soda
Tea

SPECIAL RULES FOR MIRACLE DIET NUMBER THREE

That's it.

Don't stuff yourself. You can always eat later if you're still hungry.

What does a day look like? Anything you want. For breakfast, you can have an omelette, with mushrooms and tomatoes, and a piece of cantaloupe. Hungry at mid-morning? Snack. Have an apple. Keep one on your desk at all times. Bake it with cinnamon in the microwave. Have sliced turkey. Have carrots. Is it better for you than coffee cake from the machine? Indeed.

Going out to lunch? Couldn't be easier. Grilled chicken, steamed vegetables. Grilled fish, steamed vegetables. A big salad with a chicken breast. A cool iced tea. A chicken salad at McDonald's (yes, Virginia). A chef salad, hold the cheese, bacon, and avocado.

Cooking for your family? Pick chicken, fish, or tofu for protein: happens to be better for everybody. Have a salad and a cooked vegetable, or two (instead of the potato). If you haven't tried frozen vegetables in a while, they're great. Layer eggplant and zucchini and call it lasagne. Poach the peach with berries.

MEMORANDUM TO THE FILE

Have you ever walked into one of those all-you-can-eat restaurants and thought, How can they possibly make any money here? I could easily eat my dollars' worth in my first or second go-round. But you don't. Faced with it all, you don't eat all that much—particularly if you're keeping away from what adds up fast. The all-you-can-eat restaurants stay in business the same way people lose weight on an all-you-can-eat diet. How much can you eat? How much do you want?

Start keeping track of what you eat in your nightly memo to the file. See how it looks at the end of the day. Was it a lot of food for eighteen waking hours? You're not judging, you're just observing. Someday, you're going to want to put this all together and eat like a grown-up, instead of listening to me or anyone else.

- ➤ What do you like most?
- ➤ What's been your favorite meal?
- ➤ What's your best new find?
- ➤ What's the best vegetable dish you've created?
- ➤ Have you considered soup again? Can you stand to look at it?
- ➤ What are you doing instead of eating?
- ➤ What are the hardest times of the day?
- ➤ What rituals have you developed to get through them?
- ➤ What's your best restaurant fress-out?

Remember: Any restaurant can steam vegetables, grill chicken or fish, make a salad with chicken breast, serve up a seafood cocktail, give you a bowl of vegetable or chicken vegetable soup, a green salad, a fruit salad, or just coffee, thanks, I've already eaten—and some of those beautiful strawberries.

Days 14 –18: Miracle Diet Number Four a.k.a. "Anything in Moderation"

Anything you want. Anything.

How about pancakes for breakfast with sliced peaches and maple syrup? Yum. A baked-apple waffle. A scrambled-egg sandwich. Here are some of the things you'll be eating.

Breakfast

Hot cereal with raisins and nonfat milk

Cold cereal with milk and sliced banana (aim for one-half)

Pancakes with sliced baked apple

Good girl's danish (toast with nonfat cottage cheese and cinnamon, browned in the toaster oven)

Matzo brei with applesauce

Scrambled eggs and toast

Lunch and Dinner

Turkey sandwich with lettuce, tomato, sprouts, and mustard on whole wheat, and an apple

Chicken burrito with rice and beans

Glazed orange chicken and a big salad

French bread pizza

Chicken, with steamed vegetables and white rice

Pasta with tomato and basil, and green salad

Sushi or sashimi with ginger and wasabi

Non-avocado vegetable or shrimp sushi

Pasta with chicken and vegetables

Grilled turkey burger on a low-fat bun, with grilled vegetables and a sparing amount of oil

Baked potato stuffed with vegetables, with a light cheese sauce

Charbroiled-chicken salad with low-fat dressing, and a nonfat yogurt on the way home

As for days 18 to 21, Miracle Diet Number Five, we'll get to that a little later. In the meantime, think of this diet as a contest. It is a game of skill with an unlimited number of winners. If you win, you win big. In addition to other prizes, which will be designated later by the publisher, every single winner gets a significant and real weight loss and a lasting lesson, and is prepared for a lifetime of intelligent eating. A very long lifetime, I hope.

CHAPTER EIGHT

Thinking About Miracles

The Case for Miracle Diet Number One

This is what everyone wants when they buy a diet book, and this is the very best I have found in my study and experimentation. It's hard to beat cabbage for low-calorie volume. It works. Fast. It isn't hard. That's why millions of people keep Xeroxing various versions of the cabbage soup diet every spring, and why the American Heart Association has taken to issuing warnings that this is not its cabbage soup.

It is not a diet, in the sense that a diet is a lifestyle, something you can live on. Woman cannot live on cabbage soup alone, even with fruit in the morning. But she can live on it pretty easily for three days, and learn quite a bit in the process.

What has struck me in my research is that the criticism of juice fasts and cabbage soup and all-vegetable days is not that a few such days will do you harm. Even the critics acknowledge that giving your body a break from the junk-loading might do you good. A day of cabbage and fruit is much better than a day of junk food and beer. It's that you can't live like this for very long, and that after a few days of resisting toast you'll eat a danish, and meanwhile, you won't have learned anything about how to eat right for the long run.

That's the critics' case.

Here's mine.

First, you stay on Miracle Diet Number One only for those magical first few days when your willpower is soaring and the novelty of not being stuffed with junk and the satisfaction of quick weight loss provide us the perfect opportunity to do some intensive positive casemaking and brain training. This is orientation, reminding you of what vegetables taste like and how much power you have, and making the five days that come next look like a piece of cake. (Sorry.)

Second, learning how to measure chicken portions is just one part of the brain retraining successful dieters undergo. There are other lessons that are even more fundamental. Doctors and scientists tell us that you don't need fasts to detoxify, but clearing out all the junk—and believe me, a few days of fruit and cabbage and herb tea (depending on which kind of herb tea you pick*) will clear you out—feels great. It helps you start to change your attitude toward your body, to start feeling strong and positive about who you are and the mission you are on. You know, nothing succeeds like success. Start fast and you'll keep running hard. Clichés are true.

The most important lesson you can learn eating fruit and cabbage soup is about your own power. My only rule about crash dieting is that you can't do it mindlessly; you have to think your way through it, why you're doing it, what it is about for you.

You are not a victim. Food does not control you. No one can make you eat. You don't need a bagel/muffin/cookie/danish to get through the day. When I go on fruit and cabbage soup, it's

---

*Caveat emptor: "Diet tea" or "weightless tea" often means laxative tea. Read the package instructions. If they recommend building up to the suggested dosage slowly, that's a giveaway. My husband unwittingly drank a cup and couldn't understand why he was spending so much time in the bathroom.

a declaration of independence from all the garbage that's clogged my head and my heart, literally and figuratively. I'm throwing everything out and starting fresh, and my ability to do it with ease and joy is a testament to the power that will carry you through this diet and allow you to accomplish your mission.

Remember, this is the strictest diet of all of them—and here it is, and you can do it, and not only can you do it now, but you can go back to it and do it whenever you need to, to remind yourself of your power, your control, your mission, or just to lose a couple of pounds fast when they creep back up.

But it's a crash, not an answer. You need to be able to rejoin the world.

The Case for Miracle Diet Number Two

The secret of this diet is that I've taken the basic elements of a high-protein/low-starch diet and arranged them into the five most appealing, attractive, broadly likable days I can, in the hope that it will lead you to see how well you can eat with minimal effort and great results.

The first step for most people in losing weight, the first step for me, always, after I clean out, is to up the protein and cut the starch. You know what I'm talking about. Bread. Potatoes. Pasta. Cookies. Whatever . . . But if I were to just tell you to do this, how much effort would you put into coming up with five days as varied, balanced, magically and perfectly suited to brain training as mine?

You wouldn't. You wouldn't buy fish for yourself. You might not make the salad, steam the vegetables, vary the choices, the way I have. To be perfectly blunt about it, I don't trust you to put in as much effort to take care of yourself and make this work as I'm willing to, at this stage. You're still looking for miracles, so

I'll show you one. You're still willing to take orders, so I'm going to take advantage of that. You'll eat better than you do now and lose weight because someone (me) took the time to take all those healthy ingredients and arrange them in satisfying combinations, even if they aren't magical ones. You can eat all you want of the items listed, because no one overeats chicken, or stuffs themselves with tomatoes. You don't have to worry about being hungry because you get all those celery and carrot sticks; who eats celery if they aren't hungry—and who cares if you do? Eighty percent of the calories in most salads come from the dressing, and look, the fat-free alternatives are just fine. You get lots of vegetables, because, as you are already seeing, learning to like vegetables is the key to successful dieting.

And by the time you get ready to revolt, get sick of my menu plans, have been through a "work week" of it, you'll get just what you want. Freedom. That comes first. Then responsibility.

The Case for Miracle Diet Number Three

Freedom, which thank goodness, you're finally beginning to crave. I want you to revolt. I am not your mother. I believe in responsibility. But we take it in steps. It's still my list.

One of the things that always scares me about going on a diet is the fear that I won't get enough to eat. Part of this worry is surely about being hungry, but that's only a piece of it. I use food for so many things other than hunger, after all, and I'm quite certain you do too. How do I take a break? What will I do?

That is, no doubt, why I have so many all-you-can-eat diets lining my bookshelves, from Dr. Stillman's meat-fish-eggs-and-cottage-cheese, to Dr. Atkins, who gave you all the cheese and butter and fat you wanted, to Dr. Ornish, who far more sensibly gives you none. I give myself a little.

All-you-can-eat diets appeal to the fundamental need of most of us who eat too much to know that we can. It's OK. True, no bread, no cake and cookies and treats ever on these diets, but there will be no moment in the day when you need/want/yearn for food, and can't have—something. Like a cucumber.

But all-you-can-eat diets aren't just security blankets for overeaters, or at least that's not how I think of them. They are perfectly responsible, unbelievably eye-opening learning experiences. You're not going to be wasting any calories on junk on this diet. You get your complex carbohydrates from the fruits and vegetables, protein from the chicken, fish, and nonfat cottage cheese, and bulk, bulk, bulk, from all those vegetables.

It's easy to stick to. You can eat anywhere. It's simple, straightforward, and it always works.

The secret is that no one overeats cucumber. Why would you? You can eat all you want on this diet because it's made up of low-calorie, low-fat foods that you can eat a lot of without eating too many calories; and almost no one ever does.

When was the last time you said to yourself: "I ate too many apples." Or, "I hate myself, I had so much salad." Or, "Oh, I wish I hadn't eaten that whole order of steamed vegetables."

Is there anything on my list that you have ever overeaten in its basic diet form? My guess is, no.

If there is, you should drop it, and substitute something you like less. If you really can eat six oranges in five minutes, put a limit on them or drop them from the list. I don't have mustard greens listed because I never eat mustard greens, so I don't need them on my list. By all means put them on yours. Beet greens? Why not? Butternut squash? No. That was not a mistake. I left it out on purpose and you know why. For me, it's a sweet potato.

You're in charge of making the diet work, not trying to see if you can outsmart me and eat three pounds of chicken breasts. You're not outsmarting me if you do that; you're doing yourself in. Why would you want to do that?

And I certainly didn't forget potatoes by accident. That one isn't a typo. There are a number of all-you-can-eat diets out there that are very responsible and popular and I've tried them. I've interviewed Dean Ornish on the radio and I like him enormously and highly recommend his books (and of course hope he will reciprocate). But I had a little problem with his diet, and with the Pritikin program, and I fear I'm not alone. It wasn't that it was too restrictive; that's the problem eventually and why this is the halfway point, not the end. No, the problem was more basic than that. Did someone say I could have all the sweet potatoes I want? All the potatoes? All the grains? All the corn? All the rice? All in one day? I like whole wheat pasta just fine, particularly fresser style. That's why they're not on my list. You can't have anything on the fresser list that you could easily eat a thousand calories of alone, which is what I can do in a New York minute with the potatoes/pasta/wheat/rice crowd. You're making this work, remember. No grapes. Too many calories. No dried fruit. If you don't like apples, substitute pears. Bananas aren't on my list because no one eats half a banana except a nutritionist. And a whole, big banana can easily pack 150 calories in under ten seconds.

Last year, a huge controversy erupted, at least in diet circles, about pasta. I was not the only one to discover that however the Italians may manage to pull it off, and whatever that pyramid says about six to eleven servings of grains, put a big bowl of pasta in front of me every day and I'm not losing weight anymore. The controversy was spiked by the finding that 10 percent of the public may actually have a physiological response to pasta, in terms of insulin levels, that might explain why they would gain even more weight than calorie consumption alone would explain. (How cruel can you get?)

Well, of course we all concluded that we must be allergic to pasta. Finally an answer to how I could gain weight when I'd

been so good. Here's the other half of the answer: I hadn't been
so good.

Take a wild one on a restaurant-size serving of spaghetti
with marinara sauce. It can easily hit 700 calories. You get five
ounces, not two, which is 500 calories right there, not counting
the sauce, the cheese, the glass of wine you always have with
pasta, the bite you have of your friend's veal, the half of a piece
of bread. A day's calories. Eggplant parmigiana with a side of
spaghetti is 1,200 calories, with no wine, bread, or tastes. It
doesn't matter if you're allergic. "It's the calories, stupid." They
don't disappear just because you aren't counting them.

The lesson of all-you-can-eat diets, properly structured, is ultimately the same as the lesson of all-you-can-eat restaurants.
How much do you really want to eat? The miracle is that you are
starting to ask that question for yourself.

Some people live on a diet like this forever. I do, sort of.
After a while, the good news is that you find yourself eating less
and less. The bad news is that you start getting more and more
bored. You are sick of everything. You are sick of soup, vegetables, and grilled chicken. You are ready for something different
for breakfast. Cereal would seem like heaven. This is becoming
hard work. You had lost eight pounds, but yesterday you gained
one back, and you're not telling me why, but the danger signals
are everywhere. You are bored. You are tired of being so good.
You are feeling sorry for yourself. You are sick of creating recipes
for soup and cheerfully slurping it while your children eat Oreos.
Yesterday, you had an Oreo. So there. It's time to start counting
Oreos.

The Case for Miracle Diet Number Four

Why does Sharon Stone always look so great? Reportedly,
she has a great chef who cooks healthy meals for her made of

all the things she likes. Nothing wrong with that. My friend Carrie Wiatt has built a thriving business delivering a week's worth of meals to clients' houses, many of them rich and famous, individually prepared to meet their taste and dietary needs. She does the strict portion control and the low-fat cooking techniques that allow a dieter to eat almost anything in a moderate amount, and then she delivers.

At fancy spas, you don't eat cabbage soup three times a day, or steamed vegetables for lunch every day. You eat like people do in fine restaurants, but with the magic of portion control, careful preparation, and increasingly good magic foods to work with, voilà—fettuccine Alfredo, for 250 calories instead of 1,250. This is the theory behind programs like Jenny Craig, or at least it was when I was there. You didn't give up anything; they just regulated its production and size, in the case of Jenny Craig by selling it to you. Jenny Craig beef stew, and peanut butter and chocolate bars, Salisbury steak even. When I asked the counselor what these things were doing on a diet, since it was the first time in my very long experience that I had ever met them there, she told me that many people find it much easier to eat the same things they're used to in restricted quantities than to change the way they eat.

I failed at Jenny, maybe because I don't like beef stew. But the pancakes on the Jenny Craig program were an eye-opening experience for me: you can eat a decent serving of pancakes (provided they're made with egg whites and nonfat milk, which they aren't at Carl's or Denny's, sorry), with sugar-free jam instead of syrup, and it tastes almost like the regular diner versions of my childhood. It's important to know that you can satisfy almost any craving within the limits of a diet, if you are clever about it.

OR YOU CAN BURN YOUR HOUSE DOWN COMPLETELY.

Cereal is fine, but if you have too much—and with some of them, two or three portions are easy to have—it's less fine. A sandwich at lunch is fine on a diet, but if you also hit the bread basket for dinner, good-bye, diet. What diet? A small baked potato, sure, but do you have any idea how many calories some of those steakhouse baked potatoes have? A thousand. Not counting the sour cream and chives. You'd be hard-pressed to eat that much steak.

You have been dieting long enough to hear the facts of life. If you want to eat more things, you have to start counting.

Every responsible diet book you pick up—which, unfortunately, excludes many of the bestsellers—includes the same pictures of the new government pyramid. At the bottom are bread, cereal, rice, and pasta—six servings (not for me, thank you); then vegetables, three to four servings; fruits, two to three servings; meats and poultry, fish, eggs, and nuts, two servings; milk, yogurt, and cheese, two servings; and fats, oils, and sweets, sparingly. The new pyramid was a major improvement over the last one, which was written by the cattle and dairy industry, and encouraged American families to define middle-class success by the number of nights you ate meat for dinner. The new one encourages people to think of meat as a condiment, though there has been criticism that it still doesn't go far enough. You can use it to lose weight. But you can also follow it and end up with a very high-calorie diet. Did someone really say I could have six potatoes a day, and two servings of filet mignon? That's 2,000 calories right there. Just what does "sparingly" mean? Does ice cream count as dairy? Two hundred fifty more. How about that full-fat yogurt that's so rich? Sour cream isn't a sweet. Can you have sweets sparingly and eat six potatoes a day and a steak too? Can you see why they used to hate me at the organized weight-loss programs? I should have been a tax lawyer.

The pyramid provides a starting point. On smart diets like Weight Watchers, you lose weight by being guided into making the low-fat choices in each category, which are also the lower-calorie choices. You count. You cook low-fat. You make the same sorts of choices I've been making—the white chicken, the nonfat milk, the low-fat fish—whenever you can, to leave you a little room for what you want. Two Oreos? Maybe. An extra piece of fruit? Better.

There are two steps to life in the real world, at least when you're starting out. You count servings. And just to double-check, you count calories. But wait. There's a contest coming up.

Daily Servings

Here's what the state of the common law of dieting seems to be, if you're trying to lose weight, and you're a woman. This information is distilled from the responsible diet books or at least the few that manage to be published, including ones by the American Cancer Society, the real American Heart Association, and the editors of *Prevention* magazine, with the caveat that it's my perspective being brought to bear:

Fruit: 2–3.

Vegetables: 4 plus. (There's no such thing, really, as too much cabbage unless your stomach revolts.)

Dairy: 0–2. And make it nonfat. Are we all lactose intolerant, or have we just become convinced that we are lactose intolerant? Women should take calcium supplements, since no matter what the pyramids say, most dieting women get rid of the milk first, in my observation, and on non-yogurt days, who am I to talk? Those who can, do. Those who can't, teach.

Protein: 2 plus. We've discussed this before: it is at the core of dieting theology. High-fat proteins, we now know, are bad for us, but you can lose weight on a lot of protein easier than on pasta. Chemical? Human nature? For most of us, it is simply true. I'm a high-protein, vegetable-and-fruit girl myself . . .

Oils: 0–1 (Unless you're in the Mediterranean pyramid, which allows more oil.)

Grains: The pyramid says 6–11. In my next life. Men lose weight this way. They eat a big huge bowl of rice or risotto and vegetables and fruit and they feel great, and they lose weight because they didn't eat the kung pao chicken.

When the Center for Science in the Public Interest, one of the best friends a smart dieter has (even if it doesn't always feel that way), came out with their rather disturbing findings about the calorie and fat count of average Chinese dishes, one of the points that was made repeatedly was that the Chinese eat mostly rice and a little 1,200-calorie kung pao chicken, whereas Americans tend to eat a lot of kung pao chicken and a little rice. (So that, in effect, each person gets her own 1,200-calorie order, plus rice—and then we're still hungry.) The ratios involved were 4–1, rice to chicken, for the Chinese, and just the opposite for Americans, and a number of measures of obesity and disease, including cancer, varied accordingly. So eat more rice was the message of the survey. True. If it's between rice and kung pao chicken, eat more rice. If it's between rice and steamed vegetables, eat more steamed vegetables.

My rule on grains is simple: Two is safe; above that, watch everything, and don't make mistakes around the edges. No fressing except vegetables. The right vegetables, that is.

Extras: Here and there. An empty-caloried candy bar, for 100 calories, to hit your sweet tooth at ten P.M. Does it work? Jenny Craig used to have these delicious peanut butter and chocolate bars that you could eat as an evening snack. I loved them. Plural. I found that I had a very difficult time eating only one. I would cut them up in little pieces, just like the lady said, and then I would gobble them down in multiples.

Jane Brody, whose *New York Times* food column I read religiously, says that she can have one sweet a day and do just fine, but if she eliminates that, she feels deprived, and is much more likely to overeat. My friend Pat smokes one cigarette at night. I used to eat a whole box of the Jenny Craig candy bars, not just one bar. Not good. Too many calories.

I don't think we're actually supposed to call them calories anymore. Energy. Great. You need less and less of it as you get older, or rather, you may need more, but your body has a different view. . . .

The conventional rule of thumb is that to determine how many calories a day your body needs, you take your own weight, multiply by 100, and then add 300 if you are sedentary, 500 if you're moderately active, and 700 if you're doing step between tennis games. So if you're a sedentary 140-pounder, theoretically, you need 1,700 calories a day to maintain your weight, and you will lose one pound every week (after the first drop) if you stay sedentary and eat 1,000 calories a day. A pound is 3,500 calories. Of course, that's average, and I've never met a woman with a weight problem, myself included, who wasn't sure that she had a slower than average metabolism. Maybe we all do. And prisoners of war stop losing weight; their bodies adjust, which is why if you go too low in calories, you don't get any extra weight loss from it. The old yellowed books I found on my shelf recommended that women go as low as 400 to 600 calories a day to lose weight; 900 was common. Crazy. The ones with less yellowed pages point out that adding 500 extra calories during the day (to a total of 1,000) produces the same weight loss as a 500-calorie once-a-day meal. All those poor women, myself included, who tried to do what couldn't be done, but might have done better if we'd been eating twice as much. No one who's sensible goes below 1,000.

And what do you get for that? A lot of cabbage soup, but less than one serving of a potato skin appetizer at your favorite bar.

Here's What You Get for 100 Calories

Alcoholic beverage—1 (with a no-calorie mixer—that's
   1 beer, 1 glass of wine, 1 shot of liquor)
Alfalfa sprouts—10 cups
Apple—1 medium to large (not extra large)
Apple pie—a fourth of a two-inch slice
Asparagus—20 spears
Bagel—a half of a medium-sized version; a half of a half of
   the jumbo ones
Banana—1 small, or a half of a large
Beans, refried—1/3 cup (Who eats that little?)
Beef pot pie—a fifth of a third of a nine-inch pie
Blueberries—1 cup
Brazil nuts—1/2 ounce
Bread (most kinds)—1 slice
Bread pudding—a third of 1/2 cup

Butter—1 pat (all fat)

Cabbage—5 cups raw, 3 cups cooked (the secret of the soup)

Carrots—3 to 4 large

Carrot cake—a fourth of a 3-inch wedge

Chicken, fried—a half of a drumstick

Chicken, roasted—3 ounces white meat, no skin

Chocolate—2/3 ounce (Who eats 2/3 ounce?)

Cocoa—4 cups of the diet sugar-free

Cod—3 ounces

Cookies, chocolate chip or Oreo—2 (Can you stop?)

Corn—1 ear

Corn oil—1 tablespoon

Cottage cheese, low-fat—1/2 cup (Everyone eats a cup.)

Crackers—3 normal size

Frankfurter, chicken or turkey—1, or 2 if you go fat-free

Graham crackers—3

Grapefruit—1 whole

Honeydew melon—1 1/2 cups

Mango—1 small to medium

Milk, 1% fat—1 cup (Skim has 80.)

Minestrone soup—1 cup

Nectarine—1 large

Orange—1 large

Papaya—1 medium

Pasta—1/2 cup without sauce (Figure 1 cup minimum.)

Peach—2

Peanut butter—1 tablespoon (If you can do it, more power to you.)

Pear—1

Plum—3

Popcorn (air-popped)—3 cups

Potato, baked—a half of a medium

Prunes, dried—5

Raisins—1/4 cup (Watch it!)

Raspberries—1 1/2 cups

Rice—1/2 cup cooked (That's not so much; you'll want at
least a cup.)

Roll, dinner—three-quarters of one (Fat chance, and no
butter?)

Salad dressing—1 tablespoon (Which isn't enough for anyone. The fat-free kind has 80 percent fewer calories;
give me five times as much any day.)

Sea bass—3 ounces

Shrimp—3 ounces

Spaghetti sauce—2 cups

Spinach—2 cups

Strawberries—2 cups

String beans—2 cups

Stuffing—1/4 cup (known as one taste)

Summer squash—2 to 3 cups

Tangerine—2 to 3

Tomato—3 to 4

Tuna—3 ounces, canned in water

Turkey—3 ounces, light meat, no skin

Turnip greens—3 cups

Yam—a half of a medium

Yogurt—1 cup nonfat plain, 1 small frozen nonfat,
or 1 medium frozen nonfat, sugar-free

Etc.

Some people swear by six little meals a day—each about 200
calories, a protein and a carb—and claim it's scientifically better.

The mainstream scientists disagree about the latter, sticking to that dull but seemingly accurate refrain that calories are calories, and while there are differences between fat calories and protein calories in terms of how the body uses them, it does not matter what time of day it gets them, in what order, in what combination, and so on.

Of course that doesn't solve it for me. I'm not trying to resolve a scientific dispute. I'm just interested in how to lose weight, safely and easily. Something works if it makes it easier for you to fulfill your intentions and eat what you planned. The case for six a day is that you are less hungry. The case against it is that you end up eating more—and losing less. Here's why, at least in my case. First, every time I engage in the activity of eating—particularly if we're into the world of half a potato— there will be things that I want to eat, but don't. That's just life, but facing it fully six times a day instead of three just doubles the occasions for failure. Second, if you're eating three of the six meals with other people who themselves are eating only three, or at restaurants or events catering to the common three-a-dayers, you will find it extremely easy to feel very virtuous about the fact that you're eating less than everyone else at the table. Unfortunately, you are also still eating too much. Eating three regular-size meals and three small meals is not a diet; it's a program to gain weight.

Here's an easy rule of thumb: Aim for 300 calories for breakfast, 300 for lunch, 400 for dinner, 200 for snack, and you lose weight even if you're lying to yourself a little.

Then there's the world of fat. I spent years counting fat grams, and gaining weight. The problem with counting fat grams is that the fat-free industry is at the point where you can easily gain as much weight eating fat-free as we used to do on our worst pig-out college days. Can we be honest? How do you make something taste good if it's supposed to be creamy and there's no cream? You make it sweeter. You still use the flour. The fruit juice syrup, if you use that instead, is also concentrated calories. It's fat free—but it's still a 300-calorie muffin, which is not going to do for you what a turkey sandwich would. Believe me, I have scoured the fat-free world in search of miracle solutions, but while I've found plenty of fat-free cheesecakes, they all have virtually as many calories as the real thing, and they don't even taste as good. I buy the reduced-fat Oreos for my kids because I figure they're better for us, but they are not diet food.

That doesn't mean that you should ignore fat. Far from it. I aim not to eat any, and I get plenty. If you're eating chicken and fish, there's no danger you're getting too little fat. You can take a vitamin if you're worried. What has struck me about the debate about whether you should aim for 10 percent fat in your diet (Ornish) or 30 percent (conventional, pyramid-style) is that there is no disagreement about which is better for you. Ornish wins hands down. Less is better, above zero anyway, which is not a danger most of us face. The debate is about what to tell the people. If we tell them 10 percent, will they think it is so hard— so restrictive—that they'll give up altogether, and end up getting a majority of their calories from fat, as most Americans do, a pretty horrifying thought. Conventional medicine says it's better to give people a goal they can meet than one which might exceed their grasp. If ever there were an un-American idea, that's it. Don't reach too far. Stay in the Old World.

The less fat you eat the better. Do the best you can. You don't have to be Kate Moss or Dean Ornish, but 15 percent is better than 30, and 10 percent is better than 15, and the less you eat, the less you want. Pay attention to fat to stay healthy, but for most of us, paying attention to fat alone does not make us slim.

Once you've agreed to count, you can eat anything you want. Anything at all. As long as you count it.

You have been dieting for two weeks. Your weight loss has slowed down. The crisis isn't quite so bad. Your fat pants fit again. You're looking for a new gimmick. You're bored. You need to start eating some different things, if only for a break, but you need to do it while still heading in the same direction. You need to see where alcohol is going to fit after the first two weeks, and whether you can eat one treat or not. You need to see whether bread and pasta and rice and sandwiches are going to fit, or whether they're going to push you out of the losing game. You still have more to learn before you're ready to face the world, but you're long past listening to me tell you exactly what to eat (the fresser diet ruined that) and there's danger everywhere. Free to pick anything, you might just eat everything, and go crazy and put this book back on the shelf.

So how do we get you to do this right?

There is a gimmick. This is a game. Take out a piece of paper and mark five days. Now for each day, do a perfect diet day, perfect for you, easier to stick to than mine. Easier for you. Better recipes. Yours. The greatest satisfaction for a teacher is to learn from her students. You're picking, but you have to do it now. Mr. Decina lives.

You do the menu now for the same reason countries have laws: do it in advance, and you'll do it better. Particularly if you're deciding how many pancakes you're going to eat—a fact which will also have an impact on whether you have a sandwich for lunch and pasta for supper.

Make a grid. Five days. In ink. Breakfast 1–5. Lunch 1–5. Dinner 1–5. What about snacks? What and when? Balance it now. It's too dangerous to do on the fly. You're free to use any of my meals (imitation being the purest form of flattery), you're free to go frozen or fresser, but try to give yourself at least one new test a day. How do you do with a treat? Can you have a small snack at night or does it turn huge? How do you plan to figure out what one ounce of cereal is? Do you have measures? Do you know? Buy little boxes of things, even if they are more expensive, so you'll see how little one portion really is.

Haven't you ever read a diet book and thought to yourself, hold on a minute, I could come up with a better menu plan than that. I've read hundreds in recent months, and some of them I just laugh at. This person couldn't have been an eater, I think to myself. Right? Right.

Do better. What should the next five days look like? Given that you need a burst of adrenaline right now, let's challenge your head. Just five days. Fill in the grid.

In Summation

And now what?

Let's review the course.

You can eat fruit in the morning, and all the cabbage soup you want, and lose weight. You can't live like that forever, but once you've picked your favorite recipes, you can always go back and use them when you want.

You can eat virtually all you want, so long as you limit yourself to vegetables, fruits, and lean protein, cooked without butter. You can pick or I can pick; taking care ensures that it doesn't feel like deprivation. Compared to what you're eating now, it might even feel like taking care of yourself.

You can have drinks, and treats, and pasta and potatoes, but once you do, you have to start counting. You have to figure out if you're one of those people who can eat two cookies for a hundred calories, or can't stop until you get to twenty, whether you're better off not drinking at all till you drop the weight or trying to sip one glass of wine, whether pasta moves directly from your bowl to your hips. In the process of answering those questions, you take responsibility for your diet.

By this point, whether you realize it or not, you've got it.

But have you really changed?

Let's put it to the test.

Days 18–21: Miracle Diet Number Five a.k.a. "The Grown-up Diet"

For these last three days, let's try an experiment.

Try to diet without a meal plan and a fixed set of rules. I said diet, not eat, which means not eating everything in sight. You're on a diet. You're trying to lose weight. You're aiming to weigh less. But make the decisions in the moment, and pay attention to what guides you to make the right choices. You're creating your own system.

Keep a real food journal during these three days, not just a memo to the file. Try to define a set of rules that explains the day's eating picture, the same way contestants have to figure out the questions from the answers on *Jeopardy!* What got you to this place? What system guided you? In what way did it work? Where did it fail?

If there is a miracle diet, it's in you.

CHAPTER NINE

How to Cheat

This is where most diet books end. Just do it. Good luck. It'll be just fine. Right. I know better.

Page after page about eating oranges instead of grapes is all well and good, but let's be honest. The threat to your diet is not a bunch of grapes. It is not an extra nectarine. It is a bag of cookies, a box of donuts, a croissant filled with chocolate and cream sitting on your desk eyeing you like a shiftless suitor.

You will be tested all the time. There will be moments when you honestly believe that nothing could soothe you, satisfy you, protect you, or delight you as much as a piece of cheesecake, or six, or whatever. On days when nothing goes right, there'll be no pastrami sandwich to look forward to, no pizza to eat greedily on the train, no donuts to munch in the morning, no danish, no nuts, no thank you. You will be amazed at the parade of delectable treats that pass before your eyes. Temptation will be everywhere. Terrible things will happen. Menus will speak to you. You will get cranky. You will lose your temper. You will feel tired and sluggish (or at least you'll claim you do, and blame it on lack of food). You will gain weight even when you don't cheat. Men will behave like jerks anyway.

You have to be ready to make your case at a second's notice. If you can remember nothing else, remember to always call your lawyer before you cheat. And then get ready for the fight. It is not a matter of gentle persuasion. Because it's not good enough to win some of the time, or even most of the time. Fifteen minutes can turn a day of dieting into a day of overeating.

Vic Braden, the legendary tennis coach, points out that all you have to do is return one more ball in every game than you do now and you'll reverse your won-lost percentage. One ball. That's not very much.

By the same token, it's about fifteen minutes a day that stands between a successful day of dieting and caloric catastrophe. Fifteen minutes. Maybe half an hour on really bad days. How long does it take to gobble up . . . the bread course at dinner, the last five minutes at lunch, all those last tastes for the road . . .

It's that half an hour that can do you in. My obstetrician once described his profession as endless hours of boredom punctuated by seconds of sheer and unmitigated terror; the morning before, a routine eight-hour labor in a matter of seconds became a life-or-death situation, which (because of his amazing skill) turned out fine, although he had to do a scalpel delivery, which some doctors aren't even trained to do.

Sort of like a day of dieting. You've been good for three days and now you're about to commit a major crime. This is not a problem that can be solved with techniques for low-fat cooking. They will not help you at a moment like this. The recipe for tango-mango-pie-fluff is of no use. You are in the presence of the devil. This is war.

The Case of the Chocolate Croissant

You have just had breakfast. You have resisted the donuts and the danish. The orange wasn't even sweet. The muffins looked delicious. You are way behind in your e-mail, phone messages, and paperwork, and you did not send your sister a birthday card. At least you won't have to think of food again until lunch. The grapefruit was lousy too, by the way.

You arrive at your desk and discover your basic 450-calorie chocolate croissant has been left by a "friend" as a "treat" for you. Chocolate croissants are not on the fresser diet, or any other. You know this. But you want it.

Croissant. No croissant.

You're climbing Mount Everest. It's two o'clock. Turn around.

What do you think at this critical moment?

Cheat. Lawyer. That's easy to remember.

Stop that hand. You promised at least to call your lawyer at a moment like this. This is a moment like this. You are about to commit bloody murder, and it's only nine in the morning.

Dershowitz is busy, so you'll have to do it. Here's your challenge, counselor. You have to convince yourself not to eat a single bite of that croissant. Not one. Make the full case. Hammer it until not one juror could possibly be in doubt. Remind yourself in excruciating detail just why it is you are on this diet, whom you love in life and want to be around for, whom you hate and want to get vengeance against. Let's remember those numbers on colon cancer: You cut your risk by 90 percent when you eat right. All of that arrayed against a croissant that's already stale, no better than the dozens and dozens of croissants you've had before this one, none of which have made you very happy.

Throw it away.

What do you mean, throw it away? That would be wasteful.

Eating it is suicidal. Which is worse, wasting a croissant, or using it to speed up your death, and make your hips fat?

But I deserve it.

Really. You deserve to be fat, unhappy, unhealthy, unenergetic. What terrible thing did you do to deserve that?

It's my only pleasure . . .

Is it a pleasure or isn't it? Does the good outweigh the bad, or what? If it really is your only pleasure, and you really enjoy it, why have you gotten this far in a diet book?

My friend's feelings would be hurt. Maybe the croissant has feelings too.

No one even notices. That's the truth. Your own family won't notice you're on a diet unless you tell them, or stop cooking for them. Besides, who cares? It's your health, for goodness' sake. You have a right to go on a diet.

But I've been on this stupid diet for six days and I only lost six pounds and then I gained one back and now . . .

So you think a nice big croissant will speed your weight loss? If it's hard for you to lose weight, why is that an argument for eating more? It's an argument for eating less, and exercising more.

I won't eat the whole thing.

The check's in the mail. You will eat the whole thing. You know that. You always do. Who are you talking to? How dumb do you think she is?

I won't eat later.

Please. You'll eat more later. It's a universal rule of breaking your diet that the earlier in the day you do it, the more damage you'll do.

I need something sweet to give me energy.

No, you don't. Really. You just ate. If you need energy, eat an apple. Have a turkey, lettuce, tomato, and mustard sandwich without the bread. Have something that's on your diet, not something that's off it. Remember, thin people have more energy than fat people.

Everybody else is sitting at their desks eating . . .

If everybody else at the table were shooting heroin, would you? If they were committing slow suicide, would you? Do you usually like to emulate people who are doing stupid things?

Not eating it will call attention to my weight . . .

Talking about not eating will call attention to your weight. So don't talk about it. What you eat, no one will notice. If anyone asks, which they won't, you can always say you like fresh fruit better than croissants, that you have a touch of a stomach bug, or that you've decided to live to a hundred. Say you're allergic. Lie for all I care. Just don't eat.

But there is/was nothing else to eat . . .

Not true. You just ate. You'll eat again soon. You can get healthful food everywhere. You can get a salad at McDonald's. 7-Eleven has fruit. The ice cream man has Popsicles. The mall has salad, soup, sushi, sliced turkey, steamed vegetables, baked potatoes, and black coffee. Almost every pizza place has salad. Almost every sandwich place has sliced turkey. Bars have celery. Cookouts always have fruit. Besides, so what? If there's nothing to eat that fits into the way you're eating, DON'T EAT. You are not a famished refugee. If there's nothing in a store that you really want, you don't buy something you don't want. You wait.

But it's fat-free . . .

A 450-calorie fat-free croissant still has 450 calories, at least. If you see a baked treat that is large, delicious, filling, and fat-free, it's probably loaded with calories. You tell me who splits one of those muffins into two servings? Buy low-fat snacks for your kids, not you.

But I'm hungry.

Now you don't really expect me to believe that. Eating out of hunger, well, that's practically unheard of. If you're hungry, eat an apple. Eat a slice of turkey. Eat a piece of melon. Eat a half of grapefruit. Drink a glass of water. Take a deep breath. Hungry? What a joke. Only thin people eat when they're hungry.

I've been so good . . .

So the answer is to be bad?

I've been so bad . . .

So the answer is to be bad some more?

Are you on a diet or aren't you? Do you want to be thin or fat? Do you want to fit in your clothes or not? Would you like to watch your children grow up or not? Are you going to do everything you can to live a longer, healthier life, or a shorter one in a wheelchair?

Have you thrown the croissant away yet?

When Reason Fails

Don't do it, Alan Dershowitz is screaming, you'll die young and fat and dateless. Put it down, Marcia Clark demands, you're just letting fools run your life. This is the moment when you are supposed to stop and listen to reason, when Lincoln outwits Douglas, when self-esteem replaces self-hate. At least that is what is supposed to happen. The first defense against cheating: Deliberate. Debate. Argue. Persuade. Take a deep breath. Stand tall. Win. Walk away.

Here's the problem. No one but the mythical men and women the diet doctors always parade ever sticks to any diet for any extensive period without cheating. Doesn't happen, at least so far as I've ever witnessed. Even diabetics cheat.

Moments come when reason fails, and Lincoln loses. Your boss walks out the door and you find your legs inescapably propelling you to the candy machine / coffee shop / fast-food place. Without even knowing it, you're there. Who cares if you're thin if you have to deal with a jerk like that? The train has left the station. It's on its way. It's there. What do you do?

You have a guilty client. There is only one option.

Plea bargain. Settle for a lesser offense. Do less harm.

Instead of murder, make it manslaughter. Instead of ice cream, make it yogurt. Instead of a Big Mac, a chicken sandwich. Instead of hash browns, a baked potato. Instead of lasagne, pasta with tomato. Even when you're cheating, you're choosing. Do less harm.

The less harm you do when you cheat, the less time it will take you to make up for it. That's obvious, right? Just because you're cheating doesn't mean you should be an agent of your own destruction. You're still the lawyer for losing weight. So why eat the thing that is worst for you when you're cheating, as opposed to picking the thing that will still "do" and will do less harm?

For the first year of my diet, I had a very simple rule. If you feel like cheating, head for the yogurt place. True, Häagen Dazs is better, but yogurt is good enough. One woman I know told me that her sister, who had just lost forty pounds too, sometimes ate three yogurts a day. She was shocked. I wasn't. Depending on what kind you eat, and what else you do in the day, you can easily lose weight—and certainly not gain any—on three yogurts a day. The same is not true of three Dove bars. That's the point.

Most dieters end up gaining weight because we eat much more when we're "cheating" than we would if we were just eating. It's as if there are two lights, stop and go, and since we're pushing as hard in one direction as we can when we're dieting, we turn cheating into an act of countervailing extremism. Run as fast as you can in each direction, back and forth, and you'll end up gaining a couple of pounds a year, at least.

So what do you do? You have a logical mind. Should you diet less? No, obviously not, since you're gaining weight. Or should you cheat less?

Answer: Cheat less.

How do you cheat less?

1. By making the case for yourself whenever temptation strikes. By reminding yourself about why you're on a diet, and how you want to look good, and how your clothes are already tight, and the reunion is Saturday night and your brother/father/uncle/cousin has heart problems, and you were huffing and puffing today, and your plants get better care than you do . . .

And if that doesn't work, by doing less harm when you cheat.

2. Pick the lowest-calorie "cheat" you can think of—and just eat that when you cheat, for the next three weeks. Consider it a "quasi-cheat."

Chew gum. Eat yogurt, watermelon, slushies, air-popped popcorn. Have light toast with light jam instead of a croissant. Drink the diet hot chocolate—as many as you want. Start eating

Popsicles till your tongue freezes. Buy a pack of Life Savers instead of a package of cupcakes.

Decide now what your lesser offenses will be, not as permission to cheat, but as insurance for the future. If Lincoln loses, you're still just getting popcorn.

3. Stop as fast as you can. The most dangerous thing about cheating is not what you eat when you cheat, but what happens next. Say you eat four Oreo cookies. I'm not recommending it, but it's 200 calories, not good, empty, but 200—not 2,000. The 200 calories won't ruin a 1,200-calorie day; it'll still be fine. If it started at 1,500, you'll maintain for the day. You could deal with it by cutting a fruit and adding a walk, and it would have no impact.

Or you could add another 1,800 calories because you blew it already. You could have the 900-calorie taco salad or the 1,200-calorie fettuccine Alfredo because you ate the 200 calories of cookies. Your lawyer won't like that.

When you hire Alan Dershowitz, you get a lawyer who doesn't give up. He's still arguing the case on the prison steps. He never gives up. He never says, "Since I blew it anyway, I might as well let the guy rot in jail for life." You're never supposed to say, "Since I blew it, I might as well have Häagen-Dazs." Argue for the yogurt. Push for the popcorn. Never give up.

Can you imagine yourself applying such a rule at work, or to your kids' schooling, or to anything important? If you don't do well on the first test, don't bother trying anymore. If you have a hard time at first, give up. If you make a mistake, you might as well compound it, and make lots more.

Do not stop at the bakery. Just commit a little crime.

Don't commit serial murder just because you got a speeding ticket.

Stop eating as fast as you can.

Adopt a ritual right now to end the spree. Take a walk. Say a prayer. Make a cup of tea. Stretch for five minutes. Start the day again. Say a prayer. Have an apple. Meditate.

Find something else to do.

Write a memorandum to the file addressed to the following:

When is the next reunion of your high-school class? How many years will it be? How much better do you look now? How much better would you like to look by then?

Do You Want a Watchdog?
How to Deal with Your Supportive Spouse
or Significant Other, a.k.a. the Watchdog

One of the most important things you need to discuss and decide in advance is whose diet this is: yours or ours. Does your husband need to lose weight as much as you do? Maybe so. But he's got to decide that for himself, just like you have to decide for yourself. Pushing someone to diet when they don't want to, when it's your decision, not theirs, is like giving them a gift certificate to the candy store. It doesn't work. Your husband will not get thinner this way. He will just like you less.

It is great to give support to people who are dieting—to be thoughtful when having them over, or if you're the household food shopper or dinner planner. But there's a very big difference between accommodating someone's wants and making them want what you want. Almost no one wants someone else, particularly a thin blood relative, to enforce diet rules on them. Do you?

It is extremely important to have this conversation in advance with lovers, friends, relatives, kids, or whoever else is in a position to see you eating brownies/popcorn/ice cream when you've committed not to. What do you want them to do when they see you surreptitiously reaching across the table for the bread basket, eating off the kids' plates as you clear them, wolfing down hors d'oeuvres at a cocktail party? Do you want a "Now, dear . . ." or do you want nothing said?

It used to drive me crazy when my husband would begin to clear his throat and make snide comments when I cheated. It still does, but at least I've been clear. I know when I'm cheating. I don't need anyone to tell me. I certainly don't want to discuss it with someone else while I'm doing it.

CHAPTER TEN

Making the Case for Exercise

It's like death and taxes. In every diet book, in every article about diets, in even the most irresponsible of the package inserts that come with the overpriced vitamins, there is the fine print about exercise. Just a little note to let you know, it says, that even if you believe that snake oil magically transforms fat into muscle, it still won't work unless you exercise.

The requirement that you exercise to lose weight and stay thin is absolute, unbending, and inescapable. There are some people who are thin and do not exercise. But they were born that way, and you are not one of them. If you were, you would not be reading this book. Any person who has ever bought a diet book needs to exercise to lose weight and stay slim.

I don't come to it easily. I never found a sport I was good at; never got past the initial point of frustration. I smoked cigarettes for years. I didn't jog. I never made it at aerobics classes, no matter how many gyms I joined. I had already bought and given away two exercise bicycles, which had each become dust collectors and guilt inducers rather than exercise equipment. I bought tapes and didn't watch them, books and didn't read them. When I was a kid, I hated camp. I was the worst player on the girls' softball team, in addition to being the only girl on the math team, which is why I quit them both and took up baton twirling, a skill which, you can imagine, has come in a little less handy in later life than ball playing or math might've. Athletics was the arena where I failed. By my senior year in high school, I was a steady smoker because it was cool, and my majorette's uniform was tight. I dreaded the yearly run-walk twice around the football field, something that I could do with ease today.

I now understand the problem, of course, hindsight being so clear: I never stuck with anything long enough, dared to push myself hard enough, to get past the first hurdle, the hurdle where you start knowing that you can do it, wanting to, when exercise becomes mental engagement and immediate gratification. Today, I actually like it, not only afterward, but even some of the time that I'm doing it. I like moving my body. I like feeling my muscles—pushing them, stretching them. All you have to do to get stronger is to do it. Then you get to the point where your head takes over—where it become a mental and almost spiritual challenge as much as a purely physical one. It's about focusing and breathing; about listening to your body; about feeling the difference between discomfort and pain. All that stuff the jocks say turns out to be true. You get addicted to exercise because it makes you feel better. There's even a physiological explanation for it, that relates to the release of endorphins that exercise causes. You can feel the moment when it stops hurting and your body starts celebrating the fact that it's alive. It's better than drugs. Certainly better for you.

Great, you're probably saying to yourself, because if you felt that way about exercise, you'd already be thin. The challenge is to get from there to here.

Do whatever it takes.

Bribe yourself. Reward yourself. Indulge yourself. Do anything you have to do.

It's a commitment, remember. A number of studies have

found that while you only need to do twenty minutes of aerobic exercise a day to get its benefits, those who do forty-five minutes are much more likely to lose weight—even more weight than the difference in exercise times could explain. Why? The scientists don't think it makes much sense. I think it is about the difference in heads. A twenty-minute commitment is easy to make and easier to put off; I'll find twenty minutes later in the day, you say; I'll do it instead of reading the paper in the morning, but you don't. The problem with twenty minutes is that it takes it too long to make a difference, and most of us failures never last that long. Then we stop, and start all over again at the beginning, and get no further.

It doesn't matter how you do it. It doesn't matter what you do. You have to make time in your life for aerobics and for weight-bearing exercises. You have to treat exercise as a top priority. You have to do whatever it takes. It's worth whatever it costs, if you do it. You are saving your life. It is more important than your husband's golf lessons. It is more important than new clothes, your manicure, your hairstyle, even your reading group. It's about saving your life, and also making all this effort succeed.

Remember, there should be one hour on your calendar already marked CD—RN: We're developing the health of your newest client, your most important client, the one who allows you to be and do all the things you are and do.

Take My Advice, Please

1. If you can possibly afford it, hire a personal trainer to work with you four times a week for the next three weeks. Make the dates in advance. In ink. Keep them. She shows up. You work. In Los Angeles, it would cost you $500 to $600 if you did it at home, less if you met the trainer at the gym. That's a

lot of money, I know. But let's be honest. We spend it on things with much less chance of changing us than twelve hours of hard exercise. If you look better, you won't need a new outfit. If you make twelve dates for exercise and keep them, you will have exercised twelve hours and strengthened your body that much, which is more than I can say for some of the diet places you sign up for, where you'll pay more than that for pills that could kill you and that you wouldn't need if you spent your money more wisely. Why do insurance companies only pay for sickness?

For my birthday one year, I asked my husband for a trainer. She still comes, and my husband works out with us, and we do step classes and weightlifting. Leslie charges a lot less than most "Hollywood trainers" (and is a lot better). I know a good many people can't afford that. I probably can't afford it. I shop at Ross and Loehmann's and Filene's Basement. But I also have a personal trainer. I figure I wear my body.

I am always trying to get Leslie business because she's my friend and that's how she makes her living. In the beginning, I would give women who inquired her number, but they'd never call her. It wasn't that they couldn't afford her. They just didn't call. Then we settled on a new routine. If a woman expressed enough interest to want her number, I'd give Leslie the woman's number, and she'd start calling. Sometimes, it would take four calls and three weeks; most women would tell her at the outset that their husband/boyfriend would be joining them, so it wasn't just for them, as if that would be wrong; everyone would tell her later that they thought they should have been able to get in shape on their own, and didn't really deserve a trainer.

Is that how your husband feels about his accountant? His stockbroker or financial adviser? Is that how you feel about kids' tennis lessons? Piano lessons? Is your health less important?

2. Sign up for a set of classes—for the next three weeks. Pay for them in advance. Mark them on the schedule. Buy aerobic tapes. Mark out a fast walking route. Buy an easy rider. Jog. No excuses, unless your doctor gives them. Buy an exercise bike, and close the door when you ride it. Rent videos that only you are interested in seeing. Divide them into two sessions, one day and the next, so you won't forget the story.

3. Never skip two days in a row. If you didn't exercise the day before, set your alarm for forty-five minutes earlier, and ride the bike in the morning before you go to/start to work, etc. Whatever time you normally get up, just deduct forty-five minutes. It doesn't matter how early it is. The exercise will more than make up for the lost sleep in extra energy.

If you're about to go to sleep and you haven't exercised for two days, do it now. Don't go to sleep until you exercise.

4. Make it as much fun as you can. I needed some way to exercise that I could do at home, any time of the day or night (as in, you don't go to bed until you do this). The answer was an exercise bike. I rode an exercise bike five days a week for forty-five minutes for a year. I turned it into forty-five minutes a day for *me* (how many working mothers carve five minutes a day for themselves, much less forty-five?). The key was the catalogues. I didn't exercise; I shopped. I sat on my bike and I read catalogues. I fantasized about the clothes I was going to wear when I was thin, what I liked, turning the corners over. I picked out the sheets for my son's bed. I mulled over plates. I ordered pajamas for my kids. I bought baby gifts. I also meditated, played games with the odometers and calorie meters, watched television, listened to pop music, and occasionally resorted to bribing myself by coming up with things I liked even less that I didn't have to do (for months, to my husband's chagrin, I rode the bike

rather than do my half of the taxes; there's always something even less appealing than exercise).

Give yourself permission to take a mental break when you exercise. You don't have to think about whether you've been a good enough mother, what you're going to make for supper, how you should've called your own mother, and most important, how you have so much to do that you really have no time to be riding an exercise bike. Some kinds of exercise require so much attention that you couldn't possibly think of other things. After a while, though, you may find that the key to following complicated steps or moves is precisely *not* thinking, letting your muscles remember, letting your body follow, and getting your head out of the way.

People who exercise to lose weight don't exercise as regularly as people who exercise because exercise makes them feel better. I know, we're all starting in group one here. But you have to pretend to be a group-two type, or at least give your head permission to try it on. Your body was made to move, not sit ergonomically in front of a computer screen. Maybe you were meant to be a dancer. Pretend.

5. Lift weights. Get unbelievably sexy arms and enhanced cleavage faster than you can make any changes in your thighs.

Weight training is important as you get older to fight off osteoporosis and to allow you to wave on the beach. Every responsible health institute and association tells you to do it. It also helps you lose weight: The more muscle you have, the more you can eat, because you use up more calories. It also connects you to your body in a very focused way that's new for lots of us, and definitely very sexy. How could you have missed such fun for all these years?

I started weight training six months into my diet, although in retrospect, I should've started at the beginning. And then I spent the first six months just working on my lower body, which is what always has seemed to need the most work. To be honest, I have never felt the same animosity toward my shoulders as I have to my thighs. Or, for that matter, interest. Of course, upper body is about the only place in this entire landscape that I've been able to find where women seem to hold the advantage, body-shaping wise. And most of us ignore it, until it's practically too late. Can you imagine men doing that?

The reason we have an advantage over the guys is that most women are pretty lean in their upper bodies, which means we get definition fast, much faster than on our lower bodies, even faster than the guys. Translation: Start working with dumbbells, doing simple repetitions, or working regularly on the machines at the gym, and you'll see results up top long before your hips look different. It happens quickly, and it's quite fun. I have biceps and triceps and quads and pecs, and I had them before Madonna made them sexy. They've always been sexy. I toss my suitcase into the overhead. I can carry about eight bundles at once. All you have to do to get strong is do it. I even do push-ups. They're great for cleavage. I never had cleavage before.

6. Look for chances to move. Consider them opportunities, not obstacles. Great, there's no elevator here, you can take the stairs. Great, there are no parking spaces nearby, you can park at the other end of the mall. Great, no one is home to walk the dog, you get a chance to walk around the block in the middle of working toward a deadline.

Are you done now?

Imagine that you liked to exercise. Imagine that it was a chance to do something like—eat.

Imagine that God made cheesecake low-calorie and that celery was what you had to stay away from.

It's ten o'clock at night, you've gotten the kids to bed, the kitchen cleaned, your work for tomorrow done, you've eaten your chicken salad and your grilled fish and enough vegetables to cure any disease, and there's just one little thing you haven't done: EXERCISE.

You're on, counselor. You're the lawyer for losing weight, the one who knows how to make the case at a moment's notice when she needs it, the one who is living the case. Here is the problem: Your client is exhausted, hates exercise, and has had it up to here with smart-alecky lawyers telling her what to do. It's probably just as well for Dershowitz that he's busy. I'll handle this one, Al.

Why did you clean the kitchen?

What?

Why did you clean the kitchen? You cleaned the kitchen, got your work ready for tomorrow, but you didn't exercise?

Who else was going to clean the kitchen? Would you like to have the cockroaches move in and have them elect me president of the negligent mothers' club?

Your husband, if there, could've done the dishes while you exercised. Your children, if old enough, could've done the same. If none of them exist or are old enough, you could use paper plates. Less important. And you'd be in a better mood now, and probably done better work afterward, and kissed your kids good night lovingly instead of absent-mindedly . . .

I hate exercise. The only thing I hate more than doing dishes is exercise.

Not true. You hate the idea of exercising. You probably hate the first ten to twenty minutes. But admit it. There comes a point, somewhere in there, where your body chemistry changes and so does your head. You stop worrying about whether you're going to make it through the session, because you know you will. Need I point out the lesson in that: Know it from the start.

For a very long time, my greatest fear when I'd start a new routine or take a new class was that I wouldn't be able to do it—whatever "it" was. So there I'd be, on guard for the first signs of fatigue—on the lookout for failure, utterly unaware that the first ten minutes are the hardest for everybody, and that once you get through them, you get stronger, not weaker. . . .

Has there ever, ever been a time where, after you've exercised, you regretted it?

Have you ever in your life said to yourself: "I really wish I hadn't exercised."

(I'm not talking thrill sports, we're discussing the StairMaster here.)

Is there any other activity in the entire world that you can say the same of?

Think of it this way: You don't have to feel guilty about everything else in your life when you're exercising because you're doing something important.

You have to learn to push yourself in exercise, just like you do everything else. So it's hard. So what isn't hard? It's no harder than a dozen other things you do. Just keep moving those feet up and down, riding round and round, and think about it differently. You have to approach it with an attitude of positive determination, and decide that you're doing it not because it's the only way to lose weight (which it is) but because you are going to feel so much better when you do, after you do, because the whole rest of the night will be better, the rewards will be there.

Why is this so important?

If you can think about exercise this way, you'll do it. That's the import of the studies I referred to earlier. The problem with thinking about exercise as a way to lose weight is that it doesn't offer you much at seven o'clock when you've got a sink full of dishes, screaming kids, their homework, your own work, and about as much desire to put on your gym clothes . . .

Which is why you should be wearing them already. If you come home and plan to exercise in the evening, change right into your gym clothes. No intermediate steps. You're now dressed to exercise.

If you wake up in the morning and you plan to exercise before you take your morning shower—but after car pool and walking the dog—put on your exercise clothes when you get up. Feels pretty stupid to wear them all morning and not work out.

So instead of saying to yourself, *Have I had a terrible day. And now you want me to work out, and you're telling me I have to do it or I won't lose weight but I know that I'll probably lose the same amount tomorrow morning whether I do this or not (which after the first week or so isn't much anyway), and I'm tired and it's been a long day. . . .*

You say to yourself, *Have I had a terrible day. I really need to do something that will make me feel better, stronger, calmer, clearer, and ready to face the rest of the night. What could that be? Eating a sausage sandwich? No. Yelling at the children about the mess in the house, using it as an occasion for a speech about responsibility? No.*

Let me help. How would you feel in an hour if you exercised? That good?

Look at your watch. One hour. You'll be back, a new and

better woman, in one hour. Grab the Victoria's Secret sale catalogue. Someone needs you. It's a health emergency. Mental health, too. You're looking at her.

MEMORANDUM TO THE FILE

Make yourself write it down. It's one more thing that gets you to do it, which is all it takes. What did you do? And most important, how do you feel?

After you exercise every day, take five minutes to write down how you feel—all the ways you feel better, the ways it helps you for the rest of the day. Begin to compile a list, your list, of why you actually like to exercise in the short run—not just because you need to do it to lose weight. The list is your case to exercise. Post it on the refrigerator door, on your closet door, on the television monitor, on the telephone.

Were you thinking of not exercising tonight? Open your book. Read it aloud. If you don't have sixty minutes, do what you have. Whatever you do is better than nothing. Once you start, you may even want to do more.

CHAPTER ELEVEN

Walk Like a Supermodel, Breathe Like a Yogi

Want to look ten pounds thinner and twice as self-confident, right now? Costs nothing. Legal and healthy.

How about something you can do instead of eating to deal with everything other than hunger, that has been scientifically proven to reduce blood pressure, make you healthier, happier, and spend less time in the hospital?

No-brainers, we call these.

If you think you know where I'm going, then answer this: If you're so smart, how come you're slumped like a lox in your chair, still using food to relax?

Could the problem be in your head?

I'm not a yoga teacher, or a meditation expert, and I don't pretend to be for a minute. What interests me is how you think about your body. The more you value it, the better care you will take of it. The more you appreciate it, the more you will value it.

If I gave you a brand-new car, and told you that everything was working right now, but that if it broke and couldn't be fixed, you would never get another, would you use premium fuel or would you use low-test? Would you take it for its routine maintenance, fix things promptly when they went wrong, take good care of it so it would last?

Ultimately, what makes you not want that donut is that it's lousy fuel. I'm convinced that the easiest way to diet, and maybe the only way, is to do it as part of a larger, positive, immediately rewarding effort to reconnect with your body in a beneficial way. You *know* I'm right about your body being your single biggest asset, but knowledge is not always power. What do you want me to do? My students ask me, I ask myself.

We are used to doing things. If you want to get this, you do that. Here is what I want you to do. Stand tall. Breathe deep. Do nothing.

Stand Tall

What do you think of your body?

I could tell. Anyone could, I bet, just to look at how you hold it. How do you hold something you think is precious and beautiful? With care. With pride. The way you show off pictures of your children/boyfriend/puppy.

Posture used to be something young ladies were taught. At Wellesley, they used to take pictures of the incoming freshman class standing up, naked, to chart the improvement. The practice of taking pictures was abandoned right before I got there, fortunately; unfortunately, they also stopped teaching posture.

The first time I spoke at the Reagan Library, I found myself obsessively staring at Nancy Reagan. It's not that I'm celebrity-struck. But there I was, sitting on a panel on the stage, and there she was, sitting smack in the middle of the first row, required to look interested as we yammered on about the day's topic. It wasn't the look of interest that caught my eye; I know how to fake that with the best of them. It was the way she was sitting. She looked positively regal. Totally elegant, composed. Head held high. Shoulders back. Back not even touching the chair.

Using her muscles all that time I was sitting slumped like a lox, waiting for my turn.

Standing right can take off ten pounds in ten seconds, and make you look much more fit. How much would you pay for that potion, if you could drink it? It also communicates your attitude about yourself. Are you slumping, huddled, insecure, eager not to offend? Or do you feel sexy and strong and confident, holding yourself tall, approaching the world and other people with a sense of sureness, of comfort and pride in who you are? Most corporate CEOs I meet have great posture—they walk like the football players in high school used to, carrying their bodies, not dragging them like the rest of us. You can tell models in the market by the way they walk.

In the course of the movie *Mr. Holland's Opus,* Richard Dreyfuss had to age some forty years. How does a man in his fifties play one in his twenties? As it turns out, makeup, hair color, lighting, etc.—the conventional tricks—were only a piece of the answer. Posture—standing tall, holding himself with confidence, the swagger of youth—took off as many years as the makeup. Anyone can do it.

Stand in front of a full-length mirror. Turn to the side. Trace a straight line and look at your body. Turn back to the front. Try to stand up straight with your eyes closed. Open your eyes. Now do it while you're looking.

There is an entire branch of yoga—the Alexander school— devoted to how we stand and hold our bodies. Next year, maybe. The impact on how you look is stunning. Just stunning.

Go back to the mirror. Where are your shoulders? Pull them up all the way to your ears. Now, without moving any other part of your body, just push your shoulders down. See what it feels like to lift from the abdomen while you're pushing your shoulders down and back.

I carried my shoulders next to my ears for years. I think in some strange way I thought it made me look thinner, or maybe it was just an expression of the fear I felt in the vicinity of a mirror. I still do it, even though I've been focusing on it for years. But when I don't, I look completely different.

Think of yourself as a puppet. There's a string attached to the back of your head, pulling it up. Stand sideways. Look in the mirror. Shoulders back. Chest up. That lifts your abs up and in. Now check your neck, your jaws, your teeth. Tense or relaxed? Clenched? How close together are your teeth?

Remember, if you want to check for tension, always check your jaw—we all hold it there. You'll be surprised, once you start paying attention, how often your jaw is clenched, tight, how close together your teeth tend to be. Yikes. Check your shoulders again. Still in the same place?

Look around you. How many people are sitting straight? How many are slumping? How many have their shoulders hunched up? Who looks best?

As it turns out, the easy part of posture is learning how to do it. The hard part is remembering to pay attention. That should be the goal: not to stand or sit right, but to remember to focus on it. Once you focus, you'll sit up. But how to focus?

There are all kinds of tricks, like choosing something that happens all day long—the phone ringing or starting the car—and using it as a reminder to pay attention to how you're standing or sitting, or to take a deep breath, or to close your eyes and meditate (do not do this if you are the driver, of course). I just want to add one more to the list.

When you're tempted to cheat, stand up straight. If Lincoln isn't winning, put your shoulders back. Close your eyes. Where's your chest? Remember the cheerleader in high school who used to walk with her chest sticking out?

She was right. That's where it's supposed to be.

Breathe Deep

Once you're standing or sitting properly, you can do what you probably also haven't done right since you were a baby, or at least I hadn't, until I started paying attention and taking care of my body. You can breathe. Your lungs are now in a position to expand, and get filled with what you need to survive. But my main interest isn't the biology. It's your head.

In almost any situation, particularly if you are in pain, afraid, sick, or in danger, breathing is the best thing you can possibly do. If you can breathe through labor pains, why not when a donut beckons?

Most people don't know how to breathe. Here's the test. When I say, take a deep breath, what comes out? Your chest or your abdomen?

Imagine there's a plunger inside of you. As you breathe in through your nose, the plunger inside starts going down, pushed by the air. Don't let it stop. Let the air you're taking in push the plunger all the way down, filling your lungs from top to bottom with air. As they expand, the diaphragm gets pushed down and out, so the lungs have the most room possible to expand and fill with air. Now hold it for a second. Notice what's happening. Holding yourself upright gives your lungs the most room to expand and take in air. With the diaphragm out, the plunger down, your lungs should be full—this is what full lungs feel like. It's amazing how much our bodies do for us on less.

We're born knowing how to breathe, and how much to eat. Watch babies sleeping; their stomachs go in and out. Feed babies concentrated formula, and they'll sense the difference and take less at the next meal. But then we forget, lose it, replace good habits with bad. You can't just decide one day that from then on, you're going to breathe better. It doesn't work that way. You have to practice.

There are, quite literally, exercises that will make you a better breather. They also connect you with your body, force you to sit or stand properly, calm you down, focus your energy, and make you look better. You can do them almost anywhere, and they don't even hurt. Free, too. You'd think we'd all be doing it all the time. People standing in line.

Close your eyes and breathe. Stop reading. Get comfortable. Just do it. Focus on the breath going in and out. Focus on your diaphragm. You can also do this when you're in traffic, but you must keep your eyes open. Close your eyes. Do it again. Take ten deep breaths this time. Notice what happens to your chest and shoulders. Look at yourself in the mirror. You look better. You feel better. You might really be sexy, self-assured, and supremely confident.

Say no to the peanuts. Breathe instead. Most of us eat most of the time because we desperately need something to do. Breathe.

Breathing Lessons

My three favorite breathing exercises:

The first is supposed to blow the bad stuff out. Exhale, like a sneeze, just through your nose, pulling your stomach in as you do. The rest of you stays still. That's the basic motion. Remember that the center of your body is two inches below your belly button. Now, sit tall, breathe in, and do ten fast expulsions. Inhale, exhale. Inhale and do twenty. Inhale deeply, slowly exhale, then inhale and do ten hard ones.

The second is basically holding your breath, calmly. It's supposed to nourish your body. Who knows. The trick is to inhale more deeply than usual, but not so much that you go all rigid. Inhale to a four or five count, and hold, and look at your watch, and think of getting strong, and notice how slow the seconds go by, and see if you can hold forty-five seconds. Exhale slowly, relax, and then do it again.

The third is supposed to change the air. You inhale to a five count, and exhale to a ten; inhale to a ten, exhale to a twelve. Always through the nose.

Have they cleared the breakfast trays yet? Keep breathing.

Do Nothing

I have discovered, in paying close attention to myself, that one of the reasons I eat is to do nothing. By that I mean, take a break, relax, chill out, space out, the way you are when you're standing in front of the refrigerator eating cold Chinese food or leftover pizza and thinking of nothing at all, because if you were thinking, you wouldn't be eating. For some of us, this is how we meditate. There is a very simple answer. Meditate instead.

I don't care how busy you are. The busier you are, the more you need to relax in a positive way. When you do nothing, you should do nothing—not eat.

There are hundreds of different ways to meditate, and even more books about how to do it. You probably already know how. If you don't, here's a one-minute summary, or you can check out *The Relaxation Response* from your local library. You get comfortable, close your eyes, and focus on your breath or a word or a mantra. Gently push away other thoughts. They're just thoughts, after all, they come and go, so let them go. The good ones will come back when you're thinking. Relax your body. Focus on your breath. You're meditating. That's it. Nothing.

And if you do it for twenty minutes every day, your blood pressure will go down, your health will improve, you'll be in the hospital less, recover faster when you're ill, be more productive and calmer. And this is Western medicine talking, mind you, scientific studies rather than anecdotal accounts.

But you have no time for that, do you? You have more important things to do. Name two.

Twenty minutes a day doesn't seem like much until you're trying to find time to meditate. Twenty minutes to meditate. Forty minutes of exercise to boot. Imagine spending an hour a day on yourself.

I learned to meditate the same summer I started my last diet. Coincidence? I don't believe in coincidences.

I would like to tell you that every day since then, I have found twenty quiet minutes and gone off to meditate in between writing two columns a week and raising two children and writing two books. But I'd be lying. Our TM teacher says she's meditated every day for fifteen years. That's why she's the TM teacher. But I've at least meditated enough to help me lose weight and be less crazy in the process.

Sometimes dieting can actually put you in a good mood. Those times you can handle just fine. The problem is when it puts you in a terrible mood. Food serves a lot of purposes in the day, which is why most of us eat so much of it notwithstanding our desire to be thin. Take away food and we find ourselves angry, depressed, bored, frustrated, anxious, and annoyed with nothing to chew on to distract us. This diet has put me in the worst mood, you say to yourself; what difference does it make if I'm thin if I'm walking around with permanent PMS?

This is when you need to meditate. Sure, twenty minutes is best, but no time is the worst. Two minutes is better than no minutes. Stop reading right now and do it.

CHAPTER TWELVE

Your Body, Your Rules

Welcome to Day 22. For most of us, this is where our diet ends. We manage to drop seven or ten pounds, and then it's over. The crisis passes, resolve weakens, and life isn't so much better ten pounds less. We go back to eating like we used to for a few days; or worse, we take the break as an occasion to eat everything we haven't eaten for the preceding three weeks. You put the diet book back on the shelf. Then you get on the scale and see you're down only four pounds from where you started. You keep meaning to take the book down, but other things pile up, and meanwhile since you know you're going to go back to cabbage soup any day, you eat and eat and eat. And some nights, when you're at the market, you think about buying the cabbage and the tomatoes and all that, but you end up at the fat-free baked goods aisle instead, trying to keep your brain in low gear while you buy the fat-free danish for someone else who doesn't even like it, and probably will never have a chance to eat it.

I can do it in my sleep. I did it on every diet since college until the last one.

STUPID. Absolutely, certifiably, undeniably stupid.

You are a smart woman, and you are about to do an unbelievably stupid thing.

You are not only going to reverse your weight loss, but you are undercutting yourself.

What got you this far was recognizing just how important it was, to your health, to your life, to your sense of yourself, to lose weight and get in shape.

It's no less important today, and you're not there yet, which means that eating everything in sight is the absolute and certain route to unhappiness.

You will be doubly miserable: not only will you be fat, but you will—at some point when you allow yourself to think— have to confront the fact that you failed at something that was really important.

Why are you going off your diet?

Problems. I know you've got problems. We've all got problems. One of the most interesting things I've learned about the famous people I've met is that most of them have just as many problems as anybody else and usually more; even if they make a ton of money, they even manage to have money problems.

But being fat and unhealthy and hating yourself are three additional problems that you could live without, and that solve none of the others. You'll have two more problems if you go off your diet: you'll be fat and disappointed in yourself.

Boredom. BS. Not so. I have given you the tools to diet however best suits you, and you're smart enough to figure that out. Do a different diet every day if you have a short attention span. Diversify your portfolio. Eating ice cream standing up in the kitchen is not an interesting activity. Sure, some things would taste better with cream. Couture clothes last longer and have more style, but none of us Marshalls shoppers bemoan that.

Anger. It's not fair. You were really good for three weeks, your husband dropped fifteen pounds eating just like you, now he feels great because he's just got to maintain, while you lost a measly five pounds in three weeks while you ate less and exercised more than him. Other people have a much easier time losing weight than you. There must be something wrong with the diet. Why did you waste your time and money anyway? The hell with Estrich and all of them. You're never going to eat cabbage soup as long as you live. If you're not going to look any different, you might as well eat and be happy instead of carrying stupid thermoses of cabbage soup around, and even skipping the cake at a family birthday party (which your husband didn't do, by the way).

Someday, when scientists come to understand the way the brain works, maybe they'll be able to figure out a minor adjustment for the millions of women who, like me, have specialized in the art of taking anger and turning it against ourselves. In politics, the slogan is always: Don't get mad, get even. In many of our lives, it might just as well be: Don't get mad, eat. Which might as well be: Don't get mad, get yourself.

The diet hasn't failed. You haven't failed. Five pounds in three weeks is the most I ever lost, even with no days off for cheating. That's life. A baby takes nine months to grow. Losing weight after the first week is slow for most people, particularly women, particularly women over forty. But if you could lose five pounds every three weeks, you could lose twenty in twelve weeks. Wouldn't that be great? You certainly didn't gain it in twelve weeks.

People who can lose weight quickly are generally not heavy. Life is not fair. Complain all you want. But eating is taking it out on yourself.

Look at yourself in the mirror. Is this the best you ever want to look? Are you satisfied? If not, why are you stopping?

Susan's Miracle and Victoria's Secret

My second moment of truth came three months after the first. I was in Laguna Beach with my family. I was wearing size 12 khaki shorts that I had ordered in a burst of hope from the Victoria's Secret catalogue and—surprise—they fit. With a shirt tucked in, no less. I looked like me. We were walking to a restaurant for brunch, and I was pushing my son, and remembering how I used to read ads for this particular restaurant on my radio show, and how Sunday brunch was the specialty. Crab eggs Benedict springs to mind. You get the picture.

As I walked, thanking God for my blessings, it occurred to me that all I had to do was order the fruit for lunch instead, the way I'd been doing, or maybe steamed mussels and a salad, and I wouldn't lose any ground. I could stay thin. Crab eggs who?

I had lost about twenty-five pounds by then, the most I had ever needed to lose to get back to a size 12. I'd devised a grown-up system that worked for me, with enough different variations to keep me from getting too bored, a safe crash when I got in trouble, an easy all-you-can-eat when I didn't want to pay attention; I had the making of miracles within reach, at least in their crude form. And all I had to do was keep doing what I'd been doing.

I didn't have to solve all my problems at once. The blueberry muffin demons in the kitchen could stay there. All I had to do was keep eating at the same restaurants, keep picking protein over pasta, keep studying those Victoria's Secret catalogues like the Bible code and reading diet magazines for inspiration, and I could check this piece of baggage once and for all.

Some tough things happened along the way. I got pregnant twice, sure that it was God's will, and miscarried both times.

I grieved, but I didn't eat.

I made peace with the scale. Once I realized how slow it would go, I stopped punishing myself by getting on the scale every day. I set Saturday mornings as weigh-in days, except when they fell in the wrong part of the month. Once you trust yourself to eat right, the scale will follow. It's just that it's such a slow learner that there is always a much greater likelihood that you will be disappointed by what you see than encouraged. All week long, I would imagine I had lost much more than I did, which was certainly better than feeling discouraged every morning by the silly numbers lighting up on the scale. And then on Saturday, even if I hadn't lost as much as I had, I usually had lost something and had spared myself all those other miserable days.

I'm the first to say I need a scale to keep me honest. But I don't need a daily lie-detector test, particularly when it's as unreliable as the scale is.

We all know losing weight is hard. That's why we haven't done it up until now. But in twenty-one days, you have learned that it is not impossible; that there are different ways of approaching it; that you have the power to decide what works for you and to make it work.

Some people like to visualize. Close your eyes and think about yourself, self-confident, beautiful, knowing it, doing what you like to do most, or fear most, and doing it with joy. It could happen.

If something is really important, and within your reach, why not reach? Why give up?

I heard a sermon once, in which the preacher compared life to a day at a beautiful park. In the morning you think it will last forever, but by midday, you know that time is passing, and that your moments on the pond, playing with friends, will end. That knowledge can ruin those moments by filling them with sadness or enrich them by filling them with meaning.

Life is a blessing. How you live it is your choice. Why not choose to be your best, to be happy with yourself, to be fit and strong and self-confident for however long you are blessed to be here?

Besides, you have no idea how nice it is to wake up in the morning and not think of yourself as fat and out of shape, if that's the way you thought of yourself every morning for a decade or three.

"I'm Ready!"

I grew up in the shadows of Harvard, where it's a place you dream about. I was the top girl in my high school class, but that wasn't enough for Radcliffe. I was rejected, which is how I ended up at Wellesley, which—apart from weight gain—was certainly the best place for me. But there was no doubt where I would aim for law school: to get into Harvard, to teach at Harvard, to be a tenured and full professor at Harvard and then to turn around and leave. . . .

On one of my first trips to Los Angeles to see my then boyfriend / now husband, we had dinner with a high-powered Hollywood group. "What do you do?" Someone asked me.

"I teach at Harvard," I answered. Everyone looked up.

"What grade?" one woman asked.

In Los Angeles, Harvard is a private prep school, to which Hollywood parents are very eager to send their children. The law school three thousand miles away doesn't figure much in the plans of the parents of preschoolers. No one talked to me for the rest of the night. An academic in Cambridge is a big deal. An academic in Los Angeles is more like an artist in Washington. It took me a long time to understand just what a great thing that can be.

My Harvard friends were not pleased about my departure. Many had actually sacrificed a great deal to be professors at Harvard, not to mention the kinds of compromises their careers had imposed on their spouses. In Cambridge, no sacrifice is too big for a Harvard professorship. Some of my feminist friends were the worst on the subject of my leaving. "No man would do this for a woman," they kept saying to me.

"No man would do this for a woman," I said to my friend Doe one day. I still remember her answer; like Hillel's summing up of Judaism on one foot, it is for me the insight of modern feminism.

"So what," she said.

Smart, successful women do not live their lives like men.

Why would we want to? Men don't have it all, not by a mile. Most of them don't even have any friends.

We don't live by our mothers' rules. We don't live by the boys' rules. We don't even live by each other's rules; most of us bend over backward to respect each other's decisions about careers and family, according such judgments far more deference than the usually verboten subjects of religion or politics. We live by our own rules, each one of us, within the limits imposed from the outside and the inside, we make our choices, set our goals, steer our ship. When it doesn't work, we shift course. We make it up as we go along. We don't expect someone else to take responsibility for us. We would be insulted if they tried.

I don't really know what the best diet is for you. I can distill them into types, put them in categories, lay them in sequences, use my lawyer's mind to make mine more clever than others by figuring out the underlying principles. What was stunning to me, when I laid out my diet books across the decades, was how little had changed (other than the beef and cheese), how many times I'd tried different versions of the same things. And how none of them worked as well as this last one. There were some good ones in the pile—one from a local diet center circa 1977, and another from the eighties; the now-defunct Diet Workshop and the still-thriving Weight Watchers. Then there were the not-so-good, people/places/things diets of the moment: the *Cosmo* diet guide; original editions of Stillman and Atkins; Scarsdale, Beverly Hills, Southampton.

One of them might have worked for me, if I knew then what I know now. Is mine really better? For me, maybe, but truth be told, it doesn't matter.

This isn't a contest to see who can write the best diet book. A diet is like any other relationship. You make it work or you don't. Provided you didn't make an insane choice in the first instance—a wife-beating alcoholic, meat and cheese forever—you work at it, and it works. Or you don't, and it doesn't.

Timing, one of my older married friends always said to me, when I was single and worried. (If only I'd know then that my prince would come on a later horse, I could have enjoyed the time before . . . Remember my lesson? You might as well assume . . .)

I'm ready! I would scream back. But here's the truth: If someone had fixed me up with my husband five years earlier, would we have fallen in love, or decided we had way too much in common and run in opposite directions? Timing is about your head, not the other person.

Success on a diet is ultimately about your head, not the diet.

Remember the Scarsdale diet? I still have my dog-eared copy spelling out the whole schedule, which was served in the Senate cafeteria where I worked. Assorted cheese slices for lunch on Friday. Why couldn't I have the Tuesday lunch instead? Or at least do two Tuesdays, and skip Friday altogether? I was interested to see how the late Dr. Tarnower answered the question for the millions of Americans who religiously ate cheese slices on

Friday. "In one form or another, this is probably the most frequently repeated question. While it may seem like splitting hairs to some, I think it is important to *follow the diet as written*. Your *attitude* toward a diet is an important ingredient in the success or failure of that diet for you."

I agree. I think your attitude is critical. But the attitude Dr. Tarnower and others encouraged in their mostly female patients was one of blind devotion, and I don't mean just the circumstances of his death at the hands of his jealous and mistreated lover, Jean Harris. Rules were to be followed because I say so. Ultimately, you're breeding revolution, not fostering good judgment.

Whatever diet you go on, you will get sick of it. If you can afford to go to a nutritionist every week, she'll be there when it happens, and she'll help you figure out what works and what doesn't, and how to make some changes and keep going. If you're on your own, you have to do it yourself. To do that, you have to start figuring out why it was that you were eating cheese slices on Friday to appreciate that there really was no magic, it was just a way to get you to eat a varied high-protein diet. The emperor has no clothes. There is no wizard. Thank goodness. Otherwise, how could you ever hope to do it yourself?

Guidelines for Grown-ups

In an effort to help you establish your own system that allows you, day in, day out, to expend more calories than you take in, I've compiled some tips and guidelines from grown-up dieters, just like us.

A SAFE ROUTINE

Safe choices. The same lunch. The same restaurant. A meal plan by a different name is a system.

"A turkey sandwich for lunch," my friend Susan says, without a pause, when I ask her what her secrets are. "That and fruit for breakfast, and I'm through most of the day." Unless she affirmatively wants something else, that's what she has. She likes it. She knows it works. When she gets sick of it, she'll switch to something else.

"Fruit, toast, and cottage cheese for breakfast," my friend Kath says. "Every day, perfect. Then fruit and salad for lunch, with chicken."

Grown-up dieters have restaurants they know they can always go to, snacks that are safe, meals that are time-tested as satisfying and dietetic. There was a point in my diet when I could compare steamed vegetable plates at restaurants across America, and tell you who had the best selection of salsa and mustard.

A SIMPLE SYSTEM

Categories to assess, and limit, choices instantly. No successful dieter I know reads the whole menu. You read your section. How do you get to your section? And how do you keep track?

By portion size or calories. "I'll have three hundred calories' worth," my friend Pam says, because it's lunch and that is what she consumes at lunch.

You can always start by limiting yourself to the fat-free or almost fat-free choices, which will not eliminate the muffins but will take the cheese off the pizza.

You can also avail yourself of Susan's Simple Categories:

Always: Vegetables and fruits.

Sometimes: Chicken, fish, egg whites, nonfat dairy.

Rarely: Potatoes, bread, pasta, rice, bagels, oil.

Never: Everything else, anything that has a fat-free version.

Snacks: Nonfat frozen yogurt, air-popped popcorn.

AN EFFICIENT OPERATION

Twelve hundred calories each and every day you're trying to lose weight is a tight budget to be on. You have to be careful. How do you live carefully, and make it a routine?

You can't eat what you don't buy. Always use the low-fat or fat-free version. Always make the lower calorie choice, given the option. Buy your kids the treats you like least. Never waste calories on a bad cookie or even a bad piece of fruit.

Heavy on the protein, light on the pasta. It's true. You show me a thin person who used to be heavy, and I will show you someone who considers pasta a treat. Still.

SMART SUBSTITUTES

My friend Rose tells me she just can't lose weight because she loves chocolate so. "Could you do it if you could drink all the hot chocolate you want all day?" I ask her. Her eyes open wide. *Sure.* So buy the diet hot chocolate—twenty-five calories a cup. How many cups can you drink?

If you love sandwiches, make them on forty-calorie bread instead of bagels.

If you love pizza, put some tomato sauce and fat-free mozzarella on pita or a toasted English muffin and close your eyes. If one bite will send you running for the real thing, wait till your birthday and have the real thing.

The point is that you can give up the thing you like most, or you can find a healthier way to satisfy your craving for it. Which sounds easier to you?

SELF-AWARENESS

An acceptance of individual limits. So can you eat one treat or not? How about one drink? How many days does it take you to get through a box of dry cereal? Can you control your portions, or is it easier to control what foods you eat? Every answer is fine; it's ignorance that gets you in trouble. Vary your diet. Vary your treats. Vary your exercise routines. We all get bored. Don't stay bored, and then blame it on boredom. Know when your threshold has been reached, when you need time out or a treat.

AMBITIOUS GOALS

No, not to look like you are eighteen if you're forty-eight, but to look the best that forty-eight and three kids can be, or whatever . . .

I have a new theory of why so many of us yo-yo diet, or at least why I did. It was like exercise, which I never did enough of to enjoy. In the case of diets, I never lost enough to get to a point where I affirmatively liked the way I looked. I never achieved the breakthrough that put me in another place.

"Everyone will tell you that you've lost enough," my friend Diane warned me. "Ignore them." They did. And I did. And I was right. The reason I haven't gained my weight back is not because I've lost my taste for donuts. Sadly, I haven't. It's because the pleasures of being a real size 6 are so much greater than the pleasures of donuts—far better even than being a size 10 to 12, which is only slightly better than being a 12 to 14. It's not the first twenty pounds that make the big difference. It's the last ten or fifteen, when you go from OK—at least if you wear a long sweater, or don't dry the pants in the dryer—to being able to wear whatever you want, decide what you like, get compliments for how good you look, and know that you deserve them. For the first few months, I used to just go shopping for the pure fun of trying on size 6 pants. Sheer joy. Thirty years of dreading pants shopping, squinting my eyes and holding in my stomach.

There is such a thing, obviously, as being too thin. (*Lawyer*

Alert.) But for most of us, let's be honest, it just isn't an issue. If your doctor tells you to stop, listen. If you're at or below the bottom end of the weight chart, ask him. But if you're still at the top end of the range or above it, if you're wearing your usual black leggings instead of the extra-large pair, ignore everyone and everything that's conspiring against you and just keep going.

Remember: All you have to do is what you've been doing, just keep doing it, four days out of five, nine days out of ten, just like you've been doing, and you'll be thin. It's your decision. It's within your control. If you're ever going to do it, do it now.

GENEROSITY OF SPIRIT

No one's perfect. Grown-up dieters get into trouble. But they stop, forgive themselves, and make a pot of cabbage soup.

CHAPTER THIRTEEN

Life's Little Crises

How to Fly on Airplanes

Airplanes are modes of transportation, not flying restaurants. We all know that. But something happens to most of us when we get on an airplane. It doesn't matter if we're hungry or not, if we've already had one breakfast, if it's not really dinnertime on our body clocks, if someone's meeting us with food at the other end. Get on an airplane and everyone's wondering the same thing: When do we eat? What do we eat? I have spent a good chunk of my adult life traveling on airplanes, in presidential campaigns, and in a long-distance courtship that became a commuting marriage. I think I've consumed at least a billion calories of airplane food, and other than the shrimp once on a private plane, none of it was ever memorable. In politics, where you can do six legs a day, they used to feed us on every single leg. Operating under the well-known rule that you never knew for sure when you'd eat again, I'd often eat all six. And that didn't count the snacks that were always waiting for us in the staff rooms when we landed.

Most people exercise no restraint on airplanes. The flight attendants always run out of the heaviest entree first. Lean cuisine is not what the traveling consumer wants, or so the marketing people all tell me. Sitting in an airplane is not much fun. The food is free. You can't move. It sits in front of you, usually for much longer than you'd like. Who can blame a person . . .

Before you even put down your tray, consider this:

Have you ever had a memorable plane meal?

Have you ever finished a meal on a plane and said, "Wow, that was just delicious"?

Are you hungry or bored?

Have you already eaten this meal on the ground?

Is someone meeting you to have this meal at the other end?

Is your mother cooking it for you?

Are you eating to avoid working?

If you know you'll wolf the whole thing down when the attendant puts it in front of you, DON'T TAKE THE TRAY. I believe that you have to operate on the assumption that everything placed in front of you on an airplane will end up on your thighs. If you allow them to place it there and leave it there, unless it is something you absolutely detest, you will eat it. No one has leftovers on airplanes. If you don't want it, or you don't want to eat it, don't take it.

Remember, airline food always looks better than it is. You are thirty thousand feet in the air eating a microwaved portion made en masse who knows where, who knows when. Why waste calories there? What a radical notion. Turning away free food. It is not free, if it leaves you feeling fat and sluggish and leaves your arteries coated with lard. You think that's free? They should pay you to eat that.

Some options:

Pick the healthiest choice, whether you like it or not.

Give the dessert back right away.

Ask for the whole can of diet soda.

Take a nap during mealtime.

Bring your own snacks. Throw fruit in your briefcase.

Don't accept peanuts—at least get pretzels instead.

Most important: Find something else to do. You're probably bored, not hungry. Airplanes are a fabulous place to meditate. Close your eyes for twenty minutes—you can only peek to look at your watch. Every time a thought comes to you, gently push it away and just focus on your own breathing. Everyone will assume you're asleep, but this is better. Do it during the meal service. Then have some juice or water. Who do you think feels better, you or the guy with the empty lasagne tray, the cellophane wrapper from the packaged cake, and the 900-calorie salad dressing dripping on the tray in front of him? Is this a close call?

Air travel is dehydrating. Bring a large bottle of water. Drink it. Walk to the bathroom. Stretch. Tighten your butt muscles. Do a few toe raises. Go back to your seat. Drink some more. Repeat the above. I know celebrities who always go on juice fasts on airplanes—to enforce discipline, avoid temptation. You don't need to be rich to buy juice, just remember to bring it with you.

How to Eat at Buffets

Delay eating as long as you can. Generally, the later you start, the more picked-over it will be, the less time you'll have to eat. With luck, you can practically miss dessert.

Case it. Look at the whole thing before you take a plate. I don't care if it means you'll be further behind in the line. You need to know what your choices are before you decide what to eat. The carrots and the fruit and the veggies could be anywhere. There might be rice somewhere or chopped tomatoes for the omelettes, or egg whites and Pam.

Stop. Breathe. Decide. What do you want to do? You can gorge yourself, eat everything in sight. Sound good? Think about how you'll feel in about thirty minutes. Can you be in charge for the next thirty minutes? What would you like to do for the next thirty minutes?

Are you hungry, or are you bored?

If you're hungry, consider: You can eat carrots, drink tea, make a salad, take a small portion, promise yourself a treat on the way home. (I have been known to stop for yogurt on the way home from a black-tie dinner where I didn't eat the mashed potatoes.)

Or you can eat those delicious reheated eggs that always look better than they taste, the warmed-over potatoes, the slightly stale bread that was cut in thick slices an hour before . . .

If you don't put it on your plate on the first trip, chances are you won't make an ostentatious second trip up for the forbidden item. If it's not on your plate, you won't eat it. Simple. Leave it on the serving table where it belongs.

What to Do at a Dinner Party Other Than Eat

Pamela Harriman, the wife or lover of many of the greatest, richest, most powerful men of her century, was widely regarded as one of the sexiest women of our times. Articles about her always used to refer to her milky shoulders, which was the first time I understood that there might be a breast code in news reporting. Pamela Harriman always looked good, and she got slimmer as she got older, which is the way you have to do it. But what's always struck me is that every man who has sat next to her at dinner tells exactly the same drippy story. "I know it sounds trite," one man said to me, in an apt description of how it sounded. "But when she was sitting next to you, you thought you were the most attractive, interesting, intelligent, sexy man in the room . . ." It was how she made the men feel about themselves that they always remembered. They ascribed this to what a good listener she was. Take my word for it. I sat next to some of these guys. More than listening would be required on her part for a memorable evening. She was charming, and part of her charm was that she made these guys feel like they were ten feet tall, or long. Figuring out how to make a person interesting—to themselves, and you—is a much bigger challenge than letting them bore you both. But it takes self-confidence—enormous self-confidence—to have the nerve to try.

I'd been a talk radio host for two years and a size 6 for one before I was finally secure enough to see this clearly. I'd sat next to some amazing people at dinner, and sung for my supper with the best of them. But I always felt like it was my job to produce some good story, some tasty tidbit, some worthy insight, etc. But here's the truth. Who cares what I think? Even I don't care some of the time. Most people care what they think. Our mothers taught us this, but not what to do about it. You can pretend that you think that what he thinks is fascinating. This is what my mother taught me, but I was never very good at it. Or you can make him interesting, intelligent, sexy, and charming by being that way yourself.

Believe me, it leaves you no time to eat.

Doctors

Remember. I am a lawyer. Not a doctor. A doctor should supervise your diet. I never had a doctor supervise my diet, except for the quack in Boston, but I do go for regular checkups. At least do that.

If you're overweight, it's especially important that you have a doctor you trust, because when you're overweight, you're vulnerable.

I have always associated going to the doctor—almost any doctor—with being weighed. It's the first thing they do, the first measure of you. They don't ask you what you weigh. They don't ask you to weigh yourself. You stand on the scale while a nurse weighs you.

And then everything's your fault. "Weight's high." Not only do you have something to worry about, but it's your fault.

If that's your doctor's approach, you have the wrong doctor. We all get nervous when the machines go on. One of two things is going to happen. Most likely, everything will be fine, and you'll feel great. The second possibility is that something will be amiss. That's extremely unlikely. And if it happens, thank God you'll know right now, in time to deal with almost anything. The worst thing, after all, would be to have a problem and not know it.

If the biggest threat to your health is your weight or level of unfitness, then the most important factor in picking a doctor right now is to find someone you can work with to reduce that threat. You don't need the doctor to tell you to lose weight. Presumably, you know you should. You don't even need him to explain the risks. You probably know them, and can easily research them. What you need the doctor for is to help you solve the problem.

Gas

They usually don't mention this in diet books, but you know what I'm talking about, and it's not what fuels your car.

When you start eating cabbage soup after years of processed foods, and then move on to all those raw vegetables and fruits, not to mention beans, you may find yourself feeling "fuller" than you'd like. I've been on more than one diet where it was only after a day or two that I understood what the author meant when he said you really wouldn't want to eat more. Eat? You can't button your pants or appear in polite company. What can you do?

Laugh.

First, it gets better over time, or at least that's what all the books say.

Second, it will go away. It's not as bad as being fat, which doesn't.

Third, there are things you can do. Cook vegetables, if you have a hard time digesting them raw. Eat smaller quantities in one sitting. Don't lie down after you eat. Walk around. Keep moving. Drink lots of liquids, so you'll be in the bathroom anyway. Try Prelief—an over-the-counter antacid—before the cabbage soup.

When I was nearing the end of my first pregnancy, I was told that if your water breaks in the grocery store, immediately drop a bottle of pickles, apologize, and get to the hospital.

I'm not sure what you can carry to take care of gas but your sense of humor and the knowledge that most of the time, it's just a sign that your body is doing its work of digesting some good and healthy stuff, for a change.

TEN WAYS TO AVOID OVEREATING WHEN YOU GET HOME FROM WORK

1. *Don't buy things you can't resist on the way home.*

2. *Do your nails. Let them dry.*

3. *Do not even think of entering the kitchen for the first thirty minutes.*

4. *Do not enter the kitchen at all.* Announce that for the next three weeks, dinner will have to occur as if you didn't exist—that is, entirely without your participation. You just take care of yourself. (What would they do if you were sick in the hospital? Not eat? No.)

5. *Take an extra half-hour on the way home from work and go shopping, only for yourself.* It is not necessary to buy anything; you can just try it on, which is oftentimes enough. Arrive home a little late, after they've eaten, or after you normally do, and just eat a salad or a piece of fruit and a cup of tea, and call it a day.

6. *Exercise at night.* If you can make yourself steer the wheel of your car to the gym on the way home from work, your night will be taken care of. If you tune in to your body and really work out, you can stay there afterward, and you won't need food to make you feel alive.

7. *Do things that are more fun than eating.* Go to the movies (if you can do it without gorging on popcorn); go dancing, bowling, shopping, meet girlfriends in Loehmann's instead of at a restaurant, play tennis or anything else, get your hair done, have a manicure/pedicure, a massage, a walk, a whatever. The mere act of thinking of it is good for you.

8. *Throw away everything you really like, leaving a well-stocked vegetable bin and some hot cereal.* Never go to convenience stores.

9. *Seduce someone.* Have sex repeatedly and frequently.

10. *You get to think of one.*

As a matter of fact, think of ten. Make your own list. Do it instead of eating. Do anything instead of eating. Let the moment pass. Gone.

CHAPTER FOURTEEN

Why You Need New Underwear

Smart women can be very cruel to their bodies. We fuel them poorly, do nothing to keep them in shape, constantly degrade them, and spend even our most intimate moments hiding them. "I hate my thighs," we say all the time, and we mean it. We do.

This attitude is counterproductive in any number of ways. Instead of serving as a powerful incentive to lose weight, it generally makes us feel worse, which makes us eat more, which makes us feel worse. It also enforces the sort of disconnect between the brain and the body that is exactly the opposite of what it takes to make yourself exercise every day. Look around an open dressing room and you'll see women turning away from an image of themselves, treating their body parts like pesky house rodents, brushing them aside in disgust.

I have a better idea. What if you thought of yourself as a sexy woman?

Every single survey of men and every self-help article for women comes down to the same point on sexiness. You are what you think you are. Sexy women are women who think they're sexy. They are women who like their bodies. If you think you're sexy, you are. Consider what a cycle you could be trapped in: A sexy woman is a woman who likes her body so of course she takes care of it which makes her lose weight which makes her like her body even more which makes her even sexier which makes her exercise more which makes her lose more weight . . .

"You're writing a diet book telling women to be sexy?" a journalist asks me in horror. He was apparently taught that smart women aren't sexy, that women who write about sexual abuse can't make jokes about sex, much less proclaim the value of sexuality.

I believe in sexual autonomy. If you don't want to think of yourself as sexy, you certainly don't have to. Nuns should probably skip this chapter.

For the remaining 97 percent of us who think our own version of sexiness is a goal worth pursuing on its own, and for the 2 percent who are lying when they say they disagree, the answer is most certainly yes. I think you should be sexy and smart. Both are legitimate sources of women's power if used responsibly, and illegitimate ones if abused. Both can help you lose weight and find happiness. They can reinforce each other, instead of operating at odds.

For many women in my mother's generation, all that mattered was how they looked. A woman was judged by her appearance, a man by his brains. The response of my generation was to rebel. We dressed just like the men, in our own versions of conservative suits, blouses tied in bows at our necks. We meant business. We had very little choice.

The summer after my second year in law school, a very fancy New York law firm invited me to come to their annual summer associate dinner. The idea of being invited to New York for dinner was pretty amazing to me, although in retrospect I understand: the firm literally didn't have a single woman working for them that summer, so they had me for dinner instead. I was a scholarship student, who dressed in blue jeans every day, but I decided dinner in New York deserved a new dress, particularly since I'd put on a few pounds. . . . So off I went to Filene's Basement. Twenty years later, I don't remember the name of a single person I had dinner with, but I remember what I wore: a tan dress with short sleeves, that I thought made me look thinner.

Before dinner, one of the partners took me up to the club on the top floor of the building for drinks. We had martinis. As I've mentioned, I worked my way through law school as a bartender at a working-class bar, where I learned to handle a few drinks and more than a few drunks. Good preparation for the club, I thought. So there we sat, the senior partner and I. On the second drink, he leaned over, and I learned why women wore those blouses and suits. "I thought the first woman president of the Harvard Law Review would be a real closet case," he said, looking me over carefully. "But you're a real woman."

Today, if someone said that to me, I'd laugh, and tell him that underestimating attractive women is a mistake he'll pay dearly for, and then—if I were so inclined—I'd leave him in the dust. Or at least that's what I'd like to think I'd do today. Twenty years ago, I wanted to disappear, which is precisely what a boring blue suit can do for you.

For years, I would watch my female students transform themselves to look for jobs. On interview days, they would show up in class, every trace of sexuality hidden behind long skirts, high-necked blouses, hair pulled back, desperate to be taken seriously, treated like one of the boys, looked in the eye instead of the chest. It was one thing for me to throw away my tie blouses; I had a husband and tenure, which gave me enough security to figure that anyone who didn't take me seriously could deal with it themselves. But my students enjoyed no such luxury.

Two years ago, a beautiful young woman named Tiffany

showed up for gender discrimination class in a black suit with a short skirt and no blouse underneath. She looked . . . great. It so happened that we were discussing employment discrimination that day. "Do you have an interview today?" I asked her.

"Yes," she replied.

"But you're not wearing a shirt," another student blurted out, before I could. In my day, it could be a hundred degrees outside, and you wouldn't go to an interview without anything but your bra under the jacket, much less in a short skirt, much less with the kind of jacket that barely covers your bra—if you get the picture.

"How many of you flirt in job interviews?" I asked my students. Virtually every woman raised her hand, and the ones who didn't were, to put it mildly, blown away, along with most of the men in the room.

"It's like sports," one young woman explained. "It sort of evens things out."

"I don't proposition them, for god's sake," another explained. "I just charm them, so they'll want to work with me as much as the guy who'll play tennis with them, or go to football games with them, or pitch no-hitters for the firm team."

Why not? Why not be smart and sexy? Why not enjoy your sexuality? Why not use it in the fight to lose weight?

Sexuality has always been an important source of potential power for women, a weapon that can be used as a tool of success as well as a tool of oppression. Last year, *Fortune* magazine did a cover story on the most successful women in business, and none of them were dressed in blue suits. They were frankly, intentionally, triumphantly sexy. They were, to a woman, attractive. They wore yellow suits and short skirts.

Sexuality at work is a complicated piece of business. The fact remains that more women have slept their way to the bottom than the top; there are still men who divide the world between the "closet cases" they take seriously and the "real women" they ply with martinis. You have to be comfortable with yourself. You have to be clear, and careful. (Are the lawyers happy yet? Don't harass anyone.) But having said that, I don't think there is a single woman alive who doesn't do better, personally and professionally, when she feels *great* about herself.

Is there any doubt that one of the things that has made Gloria Steinem so effective as a feminist is that she's good-looking? She is a beautiful woman and she has always presented herself in a way which highlights her attractiveness, and it increases her effectiveness. Is there something wrong with that? When I went to high school, there were the smart girls and there were the popular girls, and never the twain should meet. Because if they did, think how much they'd have going for them.

Think back to the most successful moment you've had in school or in a community group or in the work world—the day you interviewed for the big job, landed the big client, got elected chair of a committee. Do you remember what you were wearing? Do you remember how you looked? Of course you do. Do you remember how you felt about yourself? Does it make you smile? Of course it does. It does matter. It always has and always will. The question is whether it works for you, against you, or not at all.

Why not make it work for you, starting right now? If you're like most women, you're probably not as heavy as you think you are. And you know there are plenty of slightly overweight women who are unbelievably sexy (think Isabella Rossellini) and plenty of models who aren't. Maybe you're one of the Isabella Rossellini types. Maybe you're sexier than you think. Why not think of yourself that way—particularly if you are what you think, and if thinking that way will get you to exercise, and breathe, and push your shoulders down and back and lift your abdomen up . . .

No? You don't think so? You're going to tell me why I'm wrong, why you're really an unattractive, fat slob, for whom lacy underwear would be a waste of money, and thoughts of sexiness the silliness of the past? Before you do, let me ask you a question.

Whose side are you on?

Did you just switch teams, change voices?

Which case are you arguing? Do you think arguing how unsexy you are will advance some other cause? Exactly which one did you have in mind? If you hate yourself more, will you eat more or less? Will you take better or worse care of your body? What does experience suggest?

If experience suggests that tearing yourself down leads you to eat more which leads you to feel worse which leads you to tear yourself down more, could I just butt in for a second and ask why it is you would want to be on that side of the argument?

Seems to me you're on the wrong side, counselor.

You're arguing against yourself, not for yourself. You're the lawyer for losing weight, remember. The lawyer for the side that's trying to get you stuck in that vicious cycle of liking your body and thinking you're sexy and exercising and liking it more and thinking you're even more sexy and exercising even more . . . and losing all that weight in the process. Isn't that your team, too?

Imagine that Betty Bacall or Sharon Stone or Jamie Lee Curtis took over your body. What would she do different from what you do? She'd take better care of her body. She'd hold it differently, and carry it differently. She'd walk differently. She'd exercise. She'd fuel it with the high-test. Why not think about yourself differently—just for the next three weeks. Think of yourself as a woman who likes her body. Think of yourself as a sexy woman. Pretend it's you.

Indulge yourself one night. Take a bath. Buy good-smelling stuff. Think about how you feel when you're bathing a baby / your child / your puppy / your favorite handwashable item. Try to treat your own body almost as nicely. Don't tell me showers are faster. That's the point. Make time. Use lotion. A lot. Enjoy yourself. Remember, you're pretending to like yourself. Tonight, instead of settling in with a snack, put some music on—whatever you like—and dance. If you're alone, do it in your underwear, in front of the mirror. If you have kids, do it with them. It's fun to feel your body move, let it connect with the music and even let your head turn off. It's actually more fun than eating cold Chinese food. You might even forget that it's sitting in the refrigerator.

Buy new underwear. Go shopping for it. I don't care if you're on a budget. Economize on something less important and go to Victoria's Secret. Or get the catalogue and call late at night and get to know your UPS delivery people. It doesn't matter if you're going to be the only one who sees it, or notices it. It's for you. It's how you think of yourself.

How many of you expect to be partners in law firms in the next five to ten years? I ask law students in my gender discrimination class. Partnership in a law firm is the conventional and most common definition of professional success to law students who are looking ten years into the future. Every single man in the class raises his hand, along with a handful of women. What about the rest of you? I ask. Is it that the women want to pursue careers in the public interest, academics, business? Only a few. Most of them want to have children and expect to work at law firms, but in part-time or even full-time positions in which you trade family-compatible working hours for the chance of being a partner, of professional and financial success, conventionally defined.

Are they wrong? They are certainly not wrong to want the joys of motherhood, to recognize that if they are blessed with children, it is life's greatest blessing.

But you should still be able to be a partner. Why the hell not? Are all these men who are raising their hands signing up to be absentee fathers? Change the rules. Don't settle.

Sometimes I find myself in these strange partnerships of left-and-right on television against women of really great beauty, who clearly spend much more time on their hair in preparation for these encounters than I did on mine for dinner with the president. Are we now choosing female pundits for beauty, not for experience, insight, and acumen? Where are all my old friends from politics, all the women who are still eating five meals a day as they drag across the country? How come I'm never paired with good-looking men?

All true. Are we back to the days when beauty is all that counts? Did we ever really leave them?

Here's my answer. It is not an answer to all the unfairness of the world or a justification for discriminating on the basis of looks. Fight that.

But in the meantime, why not be your best? Smart and sexy. You can't stop the world from valuing these attributes, and truth be told, the world might not even be much fun if you could. So why not embrace the possibilities? And if the rules don't allow it the way you want, change the rules. Make them up for yourself. Make them work for you. Consider it your responsibility.

Recipes

I am not gifted in this regard. Not at all. As a result, there are two kinds of recipes in this book: mine, which are incredibly simple, and other people's, which are usually better and more complicated, and which might require a touch of restraint. Take your pick. The good news is that if you do choose to follow my path, Marty, my husband, will be right behind, with the last-minute doctoring instructions so you can convince people the recipe is really from a cookbook.

Before the recipes, just a few more rules:

1. Buy the best. The extra-lean turkey breast. The best vegetables you can find (preferably organic). The fancy lettuce, the imported tomato out of season. You will economize by not buying french fries, muffins, premium ice cream, grande Frappuccinos, etc. The differences matter, and make it easier. You deserve it.

2. Waste food, never calories. Don't eat your mistakes. Use the lowest-calorie alternative. Use nonstick cookware. Be sparing with the Pam. Sauté in broth.

3. Mustard. On everything. And salsa. Use low-fat salad dressing as a dip for cooked vegetables. You can make your own salad dressing in any restaurant. No one will even notice. Ask for vinegar and Dijon mustard. Pour some vinegar in a cup, add mustard, some pepper, Equal if you like, stir. It even looks like real dressing.

4. *The Goldbergs are not coming for dinner.* Just make enough for the people who regularly eat there, in the amounts they should eat.

5. *Always make two vegetables.* Then you'll have at least two things to eat.

6. *Don't feel guilty.* It's better to use fresh than frozen, pesticide-free than pesticide-full. But frozen vegetables are better than no vegetables, and canned vegetables are better than cookies. It's okay to use canned chicken stock—low-salt or no-salt—and let someone else go through the job of defatting it.

GRANDMA DOROTHY'S BETTER CABBAGE SOUP

1 large Vidalia onion, sliced
1 tablespoon canola oil
1 head green cabbage, shredded
  Kosher salt
1 28-ounce can crushed or whole tomatoes, with juice
8 cups water
1 teaspoon salt
$1/2$ teaspoon white pepper
2–3 tablespoons lemon juice (approximately 1 lemon)
2–3 tablespoons of sugar (same amount as lemon juice)
  Raisins
  Nonfat yogurt or sour cream (optional)

Sauté onion in oil in a large soup pot. Place cabbage in a colander, sprinkle with Kosher salt, then rinse well. When onion just begins to brown, add cabbage to the pot over a medium flame. Let it steam, covered, on a low flame for 20 to 30 minutes, stirring occasionally from the bottom of the pot, until cabbage is soft. Add tomatoes and juice, water, salt, pepper, lemon juice, and sugar. Toss in a handful of raisins. Bring to a boil, then lower flame and simmer for about 2 hours. Serve with a dollop of nonfat yogurt or sour cream if you like. The soup tastes even better the next day.

Susan's note: Raisins! Raisins! Buy a little teeny box if you can't control yourself with an open family-size box around the house. And remember, Grandma Dorothy had small hands. And of course, if you want to stay away from sugar, you may sweeten the soup with Equal when it's done. You may also substitute Pam for the canola oil.

SUSAN'S CARROT SOUP

First preference, cook the carrots yourself. Second preference, use frozen carrots.

The way I do it: Open a can of carrots. Open a can of low-salt, fat-free chicken or vegetable broth. Put carrots and broth in the blender with a nice couple of shakes of curry powder and some ground black pepper, and blend. Pour in a mug, and heat in the microwave.

FAST VEGETABLE PUREE

Use leftover or overcooked vegetables to make a pureed soup, the way I had to one night when I cooked the asparagus beyond recognition. "Asparagus puree," people murmured appreciatively. Served cold on a hot night, chilled in the freezer—what could be more inventive? Right.

The basic recipe:

Add whichever leftover vegetable you can no longer stand the sight of, or that overcooked mess in the pot, to fat-free low-salt chicken or vegetable broth, and puree in blender. Pour mixture in saucepan, season as you like, and simmer. If you really want to be self-indulgent, add skim milk as you simmer. For variation, add nonfat plain yogurt and/or sweetener and/or hot pepper sauce to taste. Remember: It's the vegetables, stupid.

MARTY'S SOUP DOCTORING

Here are some ways to vary the taste of Susan's basic soups:

1. Add $1/2$ teaspoon caraway seeds.

2. Add $1/2$ teaspoon cumin and a few shakes of cayenne pepper.

3. Add $1/2$ teaspoon curry powder.

4. Add 4 tablespoons cider vinegar and some Equal. For hot-and-sour soup, add cayenne pepper.

5. Puree 2 to 4 cups cooked soup in a blender and return to pot. Garnish with chopped parsley and cilantro.

6. Roast chopped onions and carrots in a preheated 300° oven, for 2 to 3 hours, or until they've turned soft and a bit caramelized. Remove from oven and add to soup pot.

QUICK COLE SLAW

Remember, cabbage is a gift from God.

1 head green cabbage
1 head red cabbage
2 carrots
1 small onion
   Miracle Whip Free (fat-free)
   Cider vinegar
   Honey mustard
   Caraway seeds
   Equal

Shred the vegetables and mix together in a large bowl. In a separate bowl, combine the remaining ingredients to make the dressing. How much of each? What looks good to you?

MARTY'S MIRACLE DRESSING

$1/4$ cup Miracle Whip Free (fat-free)
$1/4$ cup nonfat buttermilk
$1/4$ cup nonfat plain yogurt
$1/4$ cup nonfat blue cheese dressing
3 tablespoons hot-and-sweet deli mustard
1 teaspoon white horseradish
$1/4$ cup chopped fresh parsley
$1/4$ cup chopped fresh cilantro
   Coarsely ground black pepper, to taste
2–4 packets Equal

Mix all the ingredients together. Store dressing in the refrigerator. Make it last.

DANA'S MOTHER'S LOW-FAT MEAT SAUCE

$^3/_4$ *pound ground sirloin (leanest cut) or ground turkey*
breast
$^1/_2$ *medium onion, chopped*
1–2 *tablespoons olive oil (optional)*
1 *28-ounce can crushed tomatoes*
1 *28-ounce can tomato puree*
1 *tablespoon sugar*
   Kosher salt
   Black pepper
   Garlic powder
   Oregano
   Dried sweet basil

Sauté meat with onion in oil in a nonstick pot on medium heat. (You may substitute a small amount of water for the oil.) Add crushed tomatoes and tomato puree. Add sugar, and season to taste with remaining ingredients. Mix, and simmer for at least 30 minutes; 1 to 2 hours is preferable. This can be prepared a day ahead of time, and refrigerated.

JAMIE'S FAT-FREE LASAGNE

Make lasagne according to your usual recipe, but use ground turkey breast instead of beef, fat-free tomato sauce, low-sodium diced canned tomatoes, nonfat ricotta and mozzarella, and—this is Mom's secret, which kids don't like as much—layers of spinach (use the frozen kind) and even squash, so you use fewer layers of noodles. Light hand on the cheese; heavy hand on the vegetables. You can even eliminate the pasta altogether. Just remember: If fat-free lasagne weighs a ton, it probably still has a ton of calories. Just no fat.

RUTHIE'S RICE

1 6-ounce box wild rice
$^1/_2$ cup chopped pecans (optional)
6 stalks celery, chopped
4 ounces dried cherries or cranberries
$^1/_4$ cup raspberry vinegar
  Salt
  Black pepper

Prepare rice according to package directions. If using pecans, toast them in a preheated 350° oven for 5 to 10 minutes, shaking the pan once or twice to turn the nuts. Add pecans, celery, fruit, and vinegar to rice. Season to taste. This may be served warm or cold.

ISABEL'S SLOPPY BURGERS

1 pound ground turkey breast
1 onion, chopped
1 clove garlic, chopped, or 1 teaspoon garlic powder
1 tablespoon mustard
3 tablespoons ketchup or fat-free tomato sauce

Brown turkey with onion chopped by your mother. Add garlic powder if your mother didn't brown some chopped garlic with the onion. Add mustard and ketchup or tomato sauce. Spoon onto light hamburger buns (70 calories, no fat), a sliced fat-free bialy, or if you're a kid, regular hamburger buns or a sliced bagel. If you're not eating bread, serve on spaghetti squash. This is also great with a green salad.

DORA'S MOCK GEFILTE FISH

3 medium onions, 2 sliced, 1 finely chopped
6 carrots, peeled and cut in half
6 stalks celery, cut in half
4 cups water
1 teaspoon salt
$1/_2$ teaspoon white pepper
2 6-ounce cans white-meat, low-sodium diet tuna (packed in water)
2 eggs, beaten
2 egg whites
4 tablespoons matzo meal or oatmeal

Put sliced onions, carrots, celery, water, salt, and pepper into a large pot. Bring to a boil and then simmer for 20 minutes. Mix the tuna with the eggs, whites, and chopped onion. Add enough matzo meal or oatmeal so that the mixture is stiff enough to hold together. Shape with your hands into eight oval fish cakes. Gently place the cakes on top of simmering vegetables. Cover and simmer over low heat for 30 to 40 minutes. Serve with sliced cooked carrots and horseradish.

The Great Kugel Bakeoff

I never use a low-fat alternative when there's a fat-free alternative. This is one of the rules of my kitchen; it applies even during holidays. (I break it only for butter, where the low-fat alternative is really *so* much better.)

My friend Katherine, who has spent most of her life thinner than I, doesn't go quite that far, particularly when she's working from her mother's recipes. Her mother, Joy, died two years ago, but her recipes are standing the test of time. Last year, Katherine made the kugel for our Break Fast, a celebration of the end of the Yom Kippur fast, and for that reason one of my favorite meals since I started fasting at age thirteen. "I'm making it low-fat," she told me defiantly. "I will not desecrate my mother's recipe with fat-free sour cream." What could I say?

For two girls with no extended family in L.A., Katherine and I managed to invite a small army to my house, and everybody said yes. "There won't be enough kugel," she said, her panic growing.

"Not to worry," I told her. "I'll make one too." She gave me the recipe. Reluctantly.

"You're going to destroy it," she said.

"No one will complain," I told her.

The Great Kugel Bakeoff, we joked.

But whom could we get to judge? Who would have the grace, style, wit, and good taste to look at us and tell us whose kugel was really better? We would need someone of good judgment, and someone who wasn't Jewish. Anyone Jewish would surely pick the kugel that tasted most like their own mother's, regardless of how bad a cook she was. I continue to favor overbaked, dry cookies, because they remind me of my grandmother.

We hadn't solved the judging problem when the night of the Break Fast came. But luck smiled. Neighbors called to ask if they could bring a friend along. She wasn't Jewish, as it happened, which is why she was in L.A. working. No problem, I said. The more the merrier. I've got two big kugels.

That is how Katie Couric came to be the judge of the Great Kugel Bakeoff. (My own mother, by the way, was furious, particularly when she heard Katie was there. "How could you not make *my* kugel?" she asked.) We watched Katie in action, tasting each, coming up with appropriate yums, no mother's kugel to poison her judgment. Finally she rendered her Solomonic verdict. Katherine's was better, but if she hadn't tasted it, she would've thought mine simply delicious.

JOY REBACK'S LOW-FAT NOODLE KUGEL

1 pound broad or medium noodles
$1/2$ teaspoon salt
$1/4$ pound (1 stick) low-fat butter or margarine, or slightly
less (Make sure it's the kind you can cook with.)
$3/4$ pint low-fat sour cream
$3/4$ pint low-fat cottage cheese
3 eggs, well beaten
2 egg whites, well beaten
$1/2$ cup sugar or 10–12 packets Equal
3 tablespoons raisins
1 $1/2$ teaspoons vanilla
Cinnamon

Preheat oven to 350°. Cook noodles in rapidly boiling, lightly salted water until they are al dente. Drain in a colander, rinse with cold water, and drain again thoroughly.

Melt butter or margarine in a 9-by-13-inch glass or ceramic baking dish. Allow it to cool to the touch. In a large bowl, combine sour cream, cottage cheese, eggs and whites, sugar or Equal, raisins, and vanilla. Add the drained noodles. Pour into the baking dish. Mix well with your hands so that the butter is well distributed. Sprinkle the top with cinnamon. Bake approximately 50 minutes, until the pudding is golden brown.

NANA HELEN'S ALMOST FAT-FREE BLINTZES

For the wraps:
2 cups flour
$^1/_2$ teaspoon baking soda
$^1/_2$ teaspoon salt
1 cup water
2 Egg Beaters
1 tablespoon I Can't Believe It's Not Butter!, melted
   Pam for greasing

For the filling:
1 pound nonfat or low-fat cream cheese
$^1/_2$ pound nonfat farmer's cheese
$^1/_2$ pound nonfat cottage cheese
1–2 Egg Beaters

In a large bowl, mix together the flour, baking soda, salt, water, Egg Beaters, and melted butter substitute until well blended, with no lumps. Spray a small frying pan with Pam. When it's hot, spoon some of the wrap mixture onto the pan, to a diameter of about 4 inches. "Quick-fry" on one side only, then turn onto a towel to cool. Keep going until you've used up the wrap mixture and have a pile of little crepes.

In a large bowl, combine the ingredients for the filling; mix well. Place a tablespoon or two of the mixture in the middle of a wrap, tuck in the ends, then roll up.

My mother used to fry them in butter. Here are some other ideas: Microwave or bake the filled blintzes first, then brown them on high heat in the oven for a few minutes. Or "quick-fry" them in a frying pan sprayed with Pam. Another tip: Add a little pineapple or honey or other sweetener to the filling mixture, because you will miss the fat. Serve with fat-free sour cream or jelly.

GRANDMA CHAYA-SORAH'S FRUIT COMPOTE

Use fresh fruit, peeled, pitted, and sliced, or sugar-free canned fruit without syrup.

2 peaches
3 pears
3 apples
2 oranges
2 dried prunes
   A smattering of raisins
$1/2$ cup water
$1/2$ cup apple, pineapple, or orange juice
2 tablespoons sugar-free jam
   Cinnamon and cloves to taste

Put all the ingredients into a big pot and bring to a boil over a medium flame. Lower flame to simmer, and stir occasionally. Add more liquid while the compote cooks if you want it gooier. Serve hot or cold, with nonfat evaporated milk.

SUSAN'S BAKED APPLE

Core an apple. Pour some diet cherry soda or orange juice over it, and sprinkle with cinnamon. Put it in the microwave on high for a minute or two, until soft; sprinkle with Equal.

SUSAN'S CHOCOLATE SHAKE

1 can diet chocolate soda
4 ice cubes
$^1/_2$ cup skim milk

Combine the ingredients in a blender on high. Add 1 teaspoon instant coffee and call it an iced mochaccino.

ABOUT THE AUTHOR

The first woman president of the Harvard Law Review, the first woman to run a presidential campaign, and one of the nation's leading legal scholars on rape law, Susan Estrich is currently the Robert Kingsley Professor of Law and Political Science at the University of Southern California. She is a nationally syndicated newspaper columnist, a regular television commentator on legal affairs, and has been a diet maven for twenty-five years. She lives in Los Angeles with her husband and two children.